Complete Pathology

Written in partnership with the Association of Reflexologists

Second Edition 2021
First published 2011

Printed in the United Kingdom

ISBN 978-0-9553425-9-2

Essential Training Solutions Ltd.
PO Box 12565
Sawbridgeworth
Hertfordshire
CM21 1BL

+44(0)1279 726800
www.essential-training.co.uk

Disclaimer

Every effort has been made to ensure that the information and advice given in this book is accurate and up to date. Whilst the information and advice given throughout is believed to be true, safe and accurate at the time of production, Essential Training Solutions Ltd and The Association of Reflexologists cannot accept any legal responsibility or liability for any errors or omission that may be made. Essential Training Solutions Ltd and The Association of Reflexologists accepts no legal responsibility or liability whatsoever for the accuracy of the information, conclusions that may be drawn from it, how the information is interpreted and implemented by the reader or any third party, and any injury, howsoever caused, to any person. This is the basis on which the information is presented.

Contents

Abdominal Hernia 10
Achilles Tendonitis...11
Acne 12
Acromegaly...13
Addison's Disease 14
Albinism..15
Alcohol Misuse 16
Alopecia..18
Alzheimer's Disease 19
Amenorrhoea...20
Amputation 21
Anaemia (Iron Deficiency) 22
Angina 23
Anhidrosis..25
Ankylosing Spondylitis 26
Anorexia Nervosa 27
Appendicitis 29
Asthma 30
Atherosclerosis...31
Athlete's Foot..32
Atony 33
Atrophy 34
Back Pain 35
Bell's Palsy 36
Benign Prostatic Enlargement 37
Bipolar Disorder...38
Bladder Stones 39
Blisters..40
Boils..41
Bone Cancer...42
Brain Aneurysm 43
Brain Tumour..44
Breast Cancer...45
Breast Lump 46
Bromhidrosis...47
Bronchiolitis..48
Bronchitis..49
Bulimia Nervosa 50
Bunions...51
Burns and Scalds 52
Bursitis..53
Cancer..54
Candida 55
Cardiac Arrhythmia..56
Carpal Tunnel Syndrome...57
Cellulitis..58
Cervical Cancer..59
Cervical Spondylitis 60
Chilblains 61
Chlamydia...62

Chronic Obstructive Pulmonary Disorder (COPD) 63
Cirrhosis 64
Coeliac Disease 65
Cold Sore 66
Colitis 67
Colorectal Cancer 68
Common Cold 69
Concussion 70
Congenital Heart Disease 71
Constipation 72
Contact Dermatitis / Eczema 73
Corns and Calluses 74
Cor Pulmonale 75
Coronary Thrombosis 76
Cough 77
Cramp 78
Crohn's Disease 79
Cushing's Syndrome 80
Cuts and Abrasions 81
Cystic Fibrosis 82
Cystitis 83
Dandruff 84
Deep Vein Thrombosis 85
Dementia 86
Depression 88
Diabetes Insipidus 89
Diabetes Mellitus 90
Diarrhoea 91
Diverticular Disease 92
Drug Misuse 93
Dysmenorrhoea 94
Dysuria (Painful Urination) 95
Ear Problems 96
Ectopic Pregnancy 97
Emphysema 98
Endometriosis 99
Epilepsy 100
Eye Problems 101
Female Infertility 102
Fibroids 103
Fibromyalgia 104
Flatulence 105
Folliculitis 106
Foot Disorders 107
Fractures 108
Frozen Shoulder 109
Gallstones 110
Ganglion 111
Gangrene 112
Gastritis 113
Gastroenteritis 114
Genital Herpes 115
Gigantism 116

Gingivitis 117
Glandular Fever 118
Glomerulonephritis 119
Goitre 120
Gonorrhoea 121
Gout 122
Graves' Disease 123
Haematoma 124
Haemophilia 125
Haemorrhoids 126
Hashimoto's Thyroiditis 127
Hay Fever 128
Headache (Tension) 129
Head Lice 130
Heart Attack 131
Heart Disease 132
Heart Failure 133
Heartburn 134
Heel Fissures 135
Hepatitis 136
Hiatus Hernia 137
Hiccups 138
High Cholesterol 139
Hirsutism 140
HIV and AIDS 141
Hodgkin Lymphoma 142
Hydronephrosis 143
Hyperhidrosis 144
Hyperparathyroidism 145
Hypertension 146
Hyperthyroidism 147
Hypoparathyroidism 148
Hypotension 149
Hypothyroidism 150
Hysterectomy 151
Impetigo 152
Impotence 153
Indigestion 154
Inflamed Gallbladder 155
Influenza 156
Ingrown Hair 157
Ingrown Nail 158
Insomnia 159
Irritable Bowel Syndrome 160
Jaundice 161
Kidney Stones 162
Laryngitis 163
Leg Ulcer 164
Leukaemia 165
Liver Cancer 166
Lung Cancer 167
Lupus 168
Lymphadenopathy/Lymphadenitis 169

Lymphoedema 170
Lymphoma 171
Mastitis 172
Melasma 173
Meningitis 174
Menopause 175
Menorrhagia 176
Migraine 177
Modified Respiratory Movements 178
Motor Neurone Disease 179
Mouth Ulcer 180
MRSA 181
Multiple Sclerosis 182
Muscular Dystrophy 183
Myalgic Encephalomyelitis 184
Myasthenia Gravis 185
Myositis 186
Nail Conditions (Additional) 187
Nausea 190
Nephroblastoma (Wilms Tumour) 191
Neuralgia 192
Neuritis 193
Non-Hodgkin Lymphoma 194
Non-Specific Urethritis 195
Nosebleed 196
Obesity 197
Oesophageal Cancer 198
Onychia 199
Onycholysis 200
Onychomycosis 201
Osteo Arthritis 202
Osteogenesis Imperfecta 203
Osteomalacia 204
Osteoporosis 205
Ovarian Cysts 206
Paget's Disease Of The Bone 207
Pancreatic Cancer 208
Parkinson's Disease 209
Paronychia 210
Pediculosis 211
Pelvic Inflammatory Disease (PID) 212
Peptic Ulcers 213
Peripheral Neuropathy 214
Pernicious Anaemia 215
Pertussis 216
Pharyngitis 217
Pleurisy 218
Pneumonia 219
Pneumothorax 220
Poliomyelitis 221
Polycystic Ovary Syndrome 222
Postnatal Depression 223
Pre-eclampsia 224

Premenstrual Syndrome 225
Pressure Sore 226
Prolapsed Intervertebral Disc 227
Prolapse (Uterine/Vaginal)...228
Prostate Cancer 229
Prostatitis 230
Psoriasis 231
Psoriatic Arthritis..232
Pulmonary Embolism...233
Pulmonary Fibrosis 234
Pyelonephritis 235
Raynaud's 236
Renal Colic 237
Renal Failure 238
Repetitive Strain Injury (RSI) 239
Rheumatoid Arthritis 240
Ringworm 241
Rosacea 242
Sarcoidosis 243
Scabies 244
Scars 245
Sciatica 246
Scleroderma 247
Seasonal Affective Disorder 248
Sebaceous Cysts..249
Sepsis..250
Severe Acute Respiratory Syndrome (SARS) 251
Shin Splints 252
Shingles 253
Sickle Cells Anaemia 254
Sinusitis 255
Skin – Additional Characteristics and Conditions 256
Skin Cancer (Melanoma) 259
Skin Cancer (Non-Melanoma) 261
Snoring 262
Spasticity 263
Spina Bifida 264
Spinal Cord Injury 265
Spinal Disorders 266
Spinal Stenosis...267
Sprains and Strains 268
Stomach Cancer..269
Stroke 270
Sunburn 271
Superficial Thrombophlebitis 272
Sycosis Barbae 273
Syphilis 274
Tendonitis...275
Tennis Elbow / Golfers Elbow 276
Testicular Cancer 277
Testicular Lumps (Benign)..278
Tetanus...279

Thalassaemia 280
Thrush (Vaginal) 281
Thyroid Cancer 282
Tonsillitis 283
Toothache 284
Toxic Shock Syndrome (TSS) 285
Tracheitis 286
Trichomonas 287
Tuberculosis 288
Ulcerative Colitis 289
Uraemia 290
Urinary Incontinence 291
Urticaria 292
Vaginitis 293
Varicose Veins 294
Vitiligo 295
Warts / Verrucae 296
Whiplash 297
Whitlow 298
Xanthomas 299
Additional Terms 300

This page has been intentionally left blank.

Abdominal Hernia

Definition: A protrusion of tissue or organ through a weakness in the abdominal wall. The four most common types of abdominal hernia are inguinal, femoral, incisional and umbilical/paraumbilical.

Possible Causes: Any action that increases the pressure in the abdomen can cause an abdominal hernia. This includes coughing (especially if prolonged), straining from constipation, lifting heavy objects, being very overweight or being pregnant with more than one baby. Abdominal hernias are named depending on the location of the weakness in the abdomen wall. Inguinal hernia are the most common abdominal hernia and occur in the groin, particularly in men. Femoral hernia also occur in the groin and are more common women. Incisional hernia appear near old surgical scars with the weakness sometimes occurring several years after surgery. Umbilical or paraumbilical hernia appear near or in the belly button. This hernia occurs more often in pregnancy and in people who are overweight. Abdominal hernias are more likely with increasing age due to weakening muscles.

General Signs and Symptoms: Can often be asymptomatic. A bulge in the abdominal area (stomach or groin) might be visible and more noticeable when coughing or straining. This bulge can usually be pushed back in or will disappear when lying down. If the area where the hernia is becomes increasingly more painful or the bulge cannot be pushed back in, urgent medical advice should be sought.

Conventional Medical Treatment: Abdominal hernias do not always require treatment. Monitoring the hernia is usually advised if symptoms are mild or non-existent. If the location and size of the hernia could cause complications over time, surgery might be needed to repair it. Surgery involves pulling the hernia back into the abdomen and repairing the weakened muscle. This can be keyhole or open surgery.

Prognosis: Some hernia may not require treatment so can be left unless they are causing problems. Recovery from open surgery can take 4 – 8 weeks though and keyhole surgery is often much quicker.

Holistic Advice: Discover the cause of prolonged coughing. Prevent constipation by staying hydrated and eating a balanced diet with plenty of fibre. Maintain a healthy weight and lose excess weight if required. Always try to use correct lifting technique if lifting heavy weights. If this is not possible, avoid heavy lifting.

Achilles Tendonitis

Definition: Inflammation of the Achilles tendon.

Possible Causes: The Achilles tendon is the band of tissue that connects the calf muscle to the heel bone. The tendon is used when walking, running, jumping or standing on the toes. Repetitive strain or overuse of the Achilles tendon can cause it to swell via inflammation. Risk factors for developing Achilles tendonitis include age (more common as you age), being male, tightness in the calf muscles and being overweight. Running or walking on hilly terrain and wearing inappropriate or old footwear can also increase the risk of developing this condition.

General Signs and Symptoms: Common symptoms or signs include ache in the back of the leg or above the heel after exercise. Tenderness and stiffness in the area may be felt after periods of prolonged rest such as in the morning upon waking. There may be visible swelling and heat/redness from the area.

Conventional Medical Treatment: Mild tendonitis can usually be treated at home. Protecting the area from further damage and using ice packs and compression can help. Paracetamol and ibuprofen can be to treat pain and inflammation. Non-steroidal anti-inflammatory (NSAID) gel/cream can also be helpful. If the tendonitis is not going away, is severe or movement is very restricted, the person may be referred for physiotherapy. If physiotherapy is not successful then an orthopaedic specialist may offer shockwave therapy, platelet rich plasma injections or surgery to remove damaged tissue.

Prognosis: The majority of cases will resolve over time with rest. In more serious cases Achilles tendonitis can lead to rupture which may require surgical repair.

Holistic Advice: Warm up before exercise. Gradually increase distance and intensity of exercise. Ensure that footwear is in good condition and provides support.

Acne

Definition: Chronic skin disease affecting practically all adolescents.

Possible Causes: Over-activity of the sebaceous glands, which produce the oily secretion called sebum. The excess sebum secreted causes the hair follicle to block. These glands are sensitive to hormone levels and so puberty is often a common time for the disease to be triggered. In women the menstrual cycle and pregnancy can also be triggers. Stress worsens the condition, as sufferers tend to pick their spots more when under pressure. There is often a presence of micro-organisms.

General Signs and Symptoms: Sebaceous glands become blocked and infected. This leads to small spots or lumps commonly on the face, back and chest. The face is usually affected most due to the greater number of sebaceous glands.

Conventional Medical Treatment: Mild acne can be treated topically with creams and gels. In more severe cases antibiotics are used too. In extreme instances, a medication called isotretinoin can be prescribed by only a dermatologist because it can cause serious side effects and must be carefully monitored.

Prognosis: Most will have repeated episodes for several years and then the acne usually disappears. Treatments tend to be effective, taking about 2-3 months to work. Severe cases may leave scarring but prompt treatment can help to reduce this.

Holistic Advice: Requires a good skin hygiene routine using non-greasy, unfragranced, cleansing products. Wash hands before touching the face to reduce the spread of bacteria, and eat a balanced diet.

Acromegaly

Definition: A rare condition where the body produces too much growth hormone. Acromegaly is called gigantism when it develops before the end of puberty and the epiphyseal growth plates of the long bones are still open.

Possible Causes: Acromegaly occurs when the pituitary gland produces too much growth hormone. This is usually caused by a non-cancerous tumour (adenoma) on the pituitary gland. On rare occasions acromegaly is caused by a tumour in another part of the body. Acromegaly can run in families and is linked to some genetic conditions.

General Signs and Symptoms: Symptoms are wide and often develop slowly over time. Early symptoms include swollen hands/feet and numbness/weakness in the hands due to compressed nerves. Fatigue, difficulty sleeping and changes to the facial features are also early signs. As the time progresses the symptoms will become more noticeable and include abnormally large hands/feet and facial features, joint pain, fatigue and changes to the skin and vocal cords (deepening). Loss of libido, abnormal periods and erectile dysfunction may also be experienced. If caused by adenoma there may be other symptoms like headache and vision issues due to the tumour pressing on nearby nerves/structures.

Conventional Medical Treatment: Treatment dependent on symptoms. The main aim is to reduce the production of growth hormone to normal levels. This is usually achieved via surgery to remove the tumour. In some instances, the level of growth hormone may still be elevated even after surgery. If this is the case injections of medication to slow the release or reduce the effects of growth hormone will be used. If surgery and medication has not been very effective then radiotherapy can be used to target the tumour.

Prognosis: Acromegaly can be successfully treated but early diagnosis is key to reducing symptoms and any further complications. If not treated, acromegaly can lead to type 2 diabetes, hypertension, heart disease, cardiomyopathy, arthritis and polyps in the bowel.

Holistic Advice: Maintain a healthy balanced diet for wellbeing.

Addison's Disease

Definition: Disorder of the adrenal glands. Also known as primary adrenal insufficiency or hypoadrenalism.

Possible Causes: The result of the failure of the adrenal cortex to produce normal quantities of the steroid hormones cortisol and aldosterone. The most common reason is an autoimmune condition, in which the body creates antibodies that attack the adrenal cortex. If 90% of the cortex is destroyed, the adrenals are unable to produce sufficient hormones, so inducing the symptoms. Genetic composition may predispose some to autoimmune Addison's disease. Other conditions such as tuberculosis, HIV infection, some fungal infections (e.g. ringworm), genetic defect and cancer may also destroy the function of the adrenals. On occasions the adrenals may have to be removed altogether. Vitiligo, type 1 diabetes and hypothyroidism have also been linked to Addison's.

General Signs and Symptoms: Symptoms develop slowly and begin with tiredness, vague feeling of ill health, lack of energy, muscle weakness, dehydration, increased thirst, low blood pressure, increased need to urinate and a loss of appetite but a craving for salty foods. Any situation that increases the stress levels makes the symptoms worse. As the disorder progresses, or if the body is under additional stress, the initial symptoms worsen and may be accompanied by falling blood pressure on standing, dizziness, fainting, nausea, vomiting, diarrhoea, abdominal, joint or back pain, muscle cramps, exhaustion, depression and a brownish discoloration of the skin (particularly on the palms, scars, elbows, knuckles and knees). If the symptoms above are very severe it could be indicative of an adrenal crisis. This is a medical emergency and can be fatal. Although a rare condition, it is twice as common in women than men.

Conventional Medical Treatment: Corticosteroid replacement therapy is used to replace the missing hormones. This is usually taken orally but can be administered by injection. When the underlying cause is another condition, treating that will obviously treat the Addison's.

Prognosis: For autoimmune Addison's medication is permanently required, but when the condition is appropriately treated neither quality nor quantity of life should be affected. Left untreated the disease can lead to an adrenal crisis which can be fatal.

Holistic Advice: Wear a medical alert bracelet to inform medical personnel in case of an accident. Try to keep balanced and manage stress levels. Join an Addison's disease support group.

Albinism

Definition: A genetic condition that affects the production of melanin. The two main types are oculocutaneous albinism (OCA) and ocular albinism (OA).

Possible Causes: Albinism is inherited genetically. In all types of the more common OCA, the child needs to inherit a copy of the gene from each parent to have the condition. This is called autosomal recessive inheritance. In the less common OA, the condition is passed on in an X-linked inheritance pattern. If the mother carries the gene, the daughters will have a 1 in 2 chance of carrying and the sons have a 1 in 2 chance of having albinism. If the father has X-linked albinism, his daughters will become carriers and his sons will not have albinism nor will they be carriers.

General Signs and Symptoms: Albinism causes a reduction in or the complete absence of the pigment melanin that colours the skin, hair and eyes. This can cause characteristics such as very pale skin, which is prone to sunburn, and white or very light blond hair. OCA affects the skin, hair and eyes whereas OA mainly affects the eyes. A reduction in melanin can also cause eye issues due to the pigments role in developing the retina. Eye problems can include poor eyesight, astigmatism, photophobia (light sensitivity), nystagmus (involuntary side to side eye movement) and squint.

Conventional Medical Treatment: Dependent on the type and severity of the eye problem. Glasses and contact lenses may be worn and low-vision aids such a large print books, large computer screens, screen readers and magnifiers can help with reading. Photophobia can be helped by wearing sunglasses and brimmed hats outside. Squints can be treated by using glasses and eye exercises. More severe cases may be resolved through surgery or injections into the eye.

Prognosis: Albinism is a lifelong condition but it does not get worse over time. There is no cure for the eye conditions causes by albinism but low vision aids and treatments can help improve the sight. There is currently no cure for nystagmus but it does not get worse over time. Due to the lack of melanin in the skin, there is an increased risk of skin cancer.

Holistic Advice: Wear high protection SPF and be proactive with any changes to the skin.

Alcohol Misuse

Definition: When a person's alcohol consumption is harmful or they are dependent on alcohol.

Possible Causes: There are many reasons why people chose to drink alcohol. Misuse becomes a problem when a person drinks in a way that is harmful to their health and wellbeing.

General Signs and Symptoms: Short-term effects of alcohol consumption include increased heart rate, impairment to judgement/decision making and reaction time. Speech can slur and vision can be impaired. After approximately 8 – 9 units, the liver will be unable to filter the alcohol out of the body and it is likely that a hangover will be experienced in the morning (including headache, dehydration, nausea and vomiting). Excessive consumption of alcohol over a short period of time can lead to alcohol poisoning which can interfere with the bodies automatic processes such a breathing, heart rate and gag reflex. Long-term alcohol misuse over a period of years damages the organs in the body, increases blood pressure and weakens the immune system. It also increases the risk of developing many types of cancer including mouth, breast, bowel and liver cancer. Mental health may also be negatively affected. Other risks associated with both short term and long-term alcohol misuse include personal injury, violence towards others and unsafe sex. When a person loses, control over their drinking it is known as dependent drinking or alcoholism. Dependent drinkers can tolerate very large amounts of alcohol and a reduction in their intake can lead to withdrawal symptoms such as tremors, sweating, hallucinations, depression, anxiety and insomnia.

Conventional Medical Treatment: Dependent on the amount the person is drinking and whether they want to moderate (reduce) or stop (abstain) their drinking. Talking therapies, counselling (known as brief intervention) and cognitive behavioural therapy (CBT) can be offered. Information regarding alcohol support networks, keeping a drinking diary and tips about social drinking are also interventions that may be discussed. Moderation or abstinence is usually recommended when the person is regularly drinking excessively or is experiencing health problems related to their alcohol consumption. When alcohol dependent detoxing will be advised and how/where this occurs depends on the level of dependency. Medication for alcohol dependency can reduce alcohol craving, cause physical reactions to alcohol and stop the effects of alcohol.

Prognosis: Abstinence will have the greatest health benefits but moderation is often the most realistic goal. It is very important to set realistic targets under any treatment plan. Long-term alcohol misuse can have serious complications such as cirrhosis, liver disease, pregnancy complications and increased risk of many types of cancer.

Holistic Advice: Consume alcohol within guidelines. Set realistic targets under any treatment plan.

Alopecia

Definition: Loss of hair and sometimes baldness.

Possible Causes: Sudden and generally temporary significant hair loss is thought to be caused by immune system problems, anaemia, infection, stress, shock or food allergies. May occur following an illness or side effect of drugs, particularly cancer drugs. May be a sign of thyroid problems. Male-pattern baldness (see below) is caused by oversensitive hair follicles.

General Signs and Symptoms: The commonest form of hair loss is androgenic alopecia, or male-pattern baldness (although it can affect women too). The balding process is gradual, usually starting with a receding hairline. Alopecia areata involves the sudden and generally temporary loss of patches of hair and mostly affects teenagers and young adults. When the hair grows back it is fine and white before regaining its original colour. If all the hair on the scalp is lost, the condition is called alopecia totalis. If all body hair is lost, it is called alopecia universalis. Telogen effluvium is a common type of alopecia in which there is a widespread thinning of the hair, rather than the presence of bald patches.

Conventional Medical Treatment: There are drugs that can be effective to some degree in treating male-pattern baldness, but there is no effective treatment for alopecia areata. The use of steroids may help prevent hair loss and promote hair re-growth but the condition often returns when the treatment ends and there can be side effects. For extensive or total hair loss, immunotherapy, dithranol cream and UV light treatment can be used but they all carry possible serious side effects.

Prognosis: In most cases of alopecia areata the hair grows back after about a year.

Holistic Advice: Consider the whole person and identify the cause of any stress. Baldness itself can lead to stress, so the emotional needs of the person are paramount. A flattering haircut may also make a difference, and tattooing and the use of wigs can help to alleviate the obvious signs of this condition.

Alzheimer's Disease

Definition: A progressive deterioration in mental ability due to degeneration of brain tissue. It is the most common cause of dementia (the progressive loss of mental abilities).

Possible Causes: Brain cells degenerate, causing a build up of an abnormal protein that worsens the condition by destroying more brain cells. This shrinkage of the brain results in dementia. The protein also affects the brain's ability to transmit nerve impulses. The exact cause is unknown but risk factors include age, family history, Down's syndrome, having suffered whiplash or head injury and (possibly) the level of aluminium in the body.

General Signs and Symptoms: The symptoms vary from one person to another and the speed of onset can vary too. Generally the symptoms go through three stages, mild, moderate and severe. Early mild symptoms may include forgetfulness, poor concentration, confusion, difficulty saying the right words, difficulty understanding written or spoken language, and wandering and getting lost even in familiar surroundings. At this stage the sufferer is aware of the symptoms and this can lead to depression and anxiety. As the condition progresses there may be mood swings, obsessive or repetitive behaviour, personality changes, sleep problems, slow movements, unsteadiness, hallucinations and delusions. The body becomes more physically affected as the condition progresses with incontinence, difficulty swallowing, difficulty changing position and weight loss, and there is an increased risk of infection. The short term and long term memory may be completely lost. It is likely that those in the severe stage of the disease will require full time care.

Conventional Medical Treatment: The stage of the condition will be assessed with tests such as the mini mental state examination (MMSE). Various drugs can be prescribed to slow the loss of mental function. Some of the symptoms of the condition such as depression and sleeping problems may be relieved by antidepressants. A care plan will be drawn up to support day-to-day needs.

Prognosis: There is no cure, but treatment can slow the progression of the disease.

Holistic Advice: Brain function can be helped by not smoking or drinking large quantities of alcohol, taking regular exercise, eating a balanced, healthy diet, and keeping the brain stimulated by learning new skills and participating in activities.

Amenorrhoea

Definition: Absence of menstruation. There are 2 types – primary amenorrhoea, which is a failure to start menstruation, and secondary amenorrhoea, which is the absence of menstruation in a woman who has previously been menstruating.

Possible Causes: It is obviously normal not to menstruate prior to puberty, during pregnancy and breastfeeding, after the menopause or post-hysterectomy. In addition, when women stop taking the contraceptive pill it is not uncommon to have a temporary cessation of menstruation. However, at other times it may be indicative of severe weight loss, excessive exercise or an underlying disorder such as polycystic ovary syndrome, ovarian failure, thyroid or pituitary gland disorders, or eating disorders. Stress, depression, anxiety, a sudden fright or intense grief, some medications and drugs, and long-term illness may also cause hormonal disturbances that may lead to amenorrhoea.

General Signs and Symptoms: Absence of menstrual flow in women who should otherwise be having periods.

Conventional Medical Treatment: The underlying cause must be ascertained and treated. Successfully treating any underlying medical disorder will usually result in menstruation. The sufferer may be encouraged, as appropriate, to gain weight, reduce exercise and take counselling or psychological therapy. If the cause cannot be treated, hormonal treatment may be used to restart menstruation.

Prognosis: The underlying cause can usually be treated, which results in the return of menstruation.

Holistic Advice: Identifying the cause is a priority. Remember that pregnancy is contra-indicated to some complementary healthcare treatments. Try to combat stress.

Amputation

Definition: Removal of part, or all, of a limb.

Possible Causes: Amputation can occur accidentally via traumatic injury or be planned via emergency or elective surgery. Most amputations involve a section of the limb being removed rather that the whole limb. Severe infections, gangrene and serious trauma are all reasons why an amputation may take place. Primary bone cancer or soft tissue sarcoma can be treated using amputation. In some cases, deformed limbs that have limited movement or function may be removed.

Conventional Medical Treatment: Dependent on the location of the limb. Shortening and smoothing the bone above the amputated limb is often performed to allow the remaining limb to be covering adequately with muscle and soft tissue. Compression garments are often used to help reduce swelling on the stump. A physiotherapist or occupational therapist will create an individualised physical rehabilitation programme. Many amputees will have the opportunity to have a prosthetic limb fitted. The type of prosthetic recommended will depend on the type of amputation, amount of remaining muscle and the tasks the limb is required for. Prosthetic limbs are not suitable for those with ill health or who are frail due to the considerable amount of energy required to use them.

Prognosis: Dependent on the type and location of the amputation. Complications are lower in planned amputations than in emergency procedures. Feelings of depression, anxiety, grief and denial are all common and normal after amputation. Some amputees will experience pain in the stump or 'phantom limb' pain. Phantom limb pain can range from mild to severe and can be relieved with painkillers, hold/cold compresses and self-massage techniques.

Holistic Advice: Care for the stump via regular cleaning and moisturising to prevent irritation/infection. Self-massage, acupuncture and TENS machines are thought to be helpful for pain.

Anaemia (Iron Deficiency)

Definition: Deficiency or abnormality of haemoglobin.

Possible Causes: There are several types of anaemia. Iron deficiency is by far the most common. Iron is required for the body to make haemoglobin, which stores and transports oxygen. An iron deficiency impairs the body's ability to make haemoglobin resulting in anaemia. There are many causes of iron deficiency including bleeding from the digestive tract, heavy menstrual bleeding, pregnancy, trauma resulting in blood loss, a variety of medical conditions, a lack of iron in the diet and malabsorption problems. The prolonged use of aspirin and nonsteroidal anti-inflammatory drugs can cause bleeding from the stomach lining. The causes of other types of anaemia include a lack of vitamin B12 or folic acid, inherited abnormalities of haemoglobin, the excessive rapid destruction of red blood cells and the failure to produce sufficient red blood cells.

General Signs and Symptoms: The condition may develop slowly showing symptoms such as tiredness, lethargy, weakness, shortness of breath, palpitations, headache, faintness, fading complexion, pale colour on inside of eyelids, brittle nails, cracks in the skin at the sides of the mouth, smooth tongue and an increased respiratory rate.

Conventional Medical Treatment: Establishing the underlying cause is a priority so it can be treated. The iron levels in the body can be restored using iron supplements and an iron-rich diet. The iron level should be monitored regularly. In extreme cases a blood transfusion may be necessary.

Prognosis: Establishing and treating the cause and raising the iron levels should cure the anaemia. Serious or long-term problems are rare.

Holistic Advice: Eat red meat, dried fruit and iron-rich vegetables regularly. Reduce tea and coffee intake. Seek dietary advice.

Angina

Definition: A syndrome caused by a restriction of the blood supply to the heart. There are 2 types, stable and unstable. In stable angina the symptoms are brought on by exercise, subside at rest, and usually develop gradually over time. In unstable angina the symptoms develop rapidly and can persist at rest.

Possible Causes: Angina is indicative of an inadequate blood supply to the heart muscle. Stable angina is commonly due to coronary heart disease in which the coronary arteries harden and narrow (atherosclerosis), reducing their ability to supply blood. At rest the supply may be sufficient, but during exercise or stress the heart may receive an insufficient supply of blood which triggers the syndrome. Unstable angina can be caused by the rupture of the fatty deposits in the arteries which then interfere with the blood flow causing blood clots. The blood clots can quickly grow, reducing the blood supply to the heart. Risk factors for angina include a high fat diet, a high cholesterol level, smoking, hypertension, diabetes, age, obesity, high alcohol consumption and family history. Less commonly angina can be caused by a temporary spasm of the coronary arteries, damaged heart valves and anaemia.

General Signs and Symptoms: An attack of stable angina is typified by pain or discomfort in the chest, often radiating to the neck, jaw and down the left arm. There may be sweating, breathlessness, belching and nausea. It is usually triggered by exercise but can be aggravated by exposure to cold or immediately after eating a meal. The symptoms subside during rest. The symptoms of unstable angina are the same, but they can develop without the usual triggers, last for longer, and can persist at rest. Attacks of unstable angina may not respond to the usual treatment and should be treated as a medical emergency.

Conventional Medical Treatment: For stable angina a wide range of medication is used to relieve symptoms during an attack (e.g. glycerol trinitrate spray or tablets), help prevent further attacks (e.g. beta blockers) and reduce the chance of a heart attack or stroke (e.g. statins). Surgical techniques such as coronary angioplasty (to widen the narrowing) and artery bypass grafts (to bypass the restriction) can be used. For unstable angina the emergency treatment focuses on preventing blood clots forming using blood-thinning drugs. The medication/surgery required is then established.

Prognosis: The outlook depends on the extent of coronary heart disease and the presence of other factors such as hypertension and additional chronic conditions. Taking the correct balance of medications and making lifestyle changes can improve the prognosis. Coronary heart disease carries an increased risk of a heart attack or stroke.

Holistic Advice: Lifestyle changes are very important to prevent the condition or to prevent the condition from worsening. Stop smoking and lose any excess weight. Take regular exercise and reduce stress levels. Maintain a healthy low fat, high fibre diet. Many people with coronary heart disease live in fear of a heart attack, feel hopeless, out of control and depressed, so address these issues in any complementary healthcare treatment. Support groups can be of use. Any unexplained chest pains that a client reports to you requires you to inform them to seek medical attention.

Anhidrosis

Definition: The inability to sweat.

Possible Causes: Occurs when the sweat glands do not function as they should. This can be due to a number of conditions that affect the nerves or skin such as diabetes, psoriasis and Guillain-Barré syndrome. Damage to the skin from trauma and some medications can also cause issues with the sweat glands. Dehydration and heat stroke are causes of anhidrosis that can happen to anyone without underlying medical conditions.

General Signs and Symptoms: Can be difficult to detect as the lack of sweat production may be localised to one area, in patches or across the whole body. Aside from little to no sweat production there may be dizziness, muscles cramps, feeling hot and flushing.

Conventional Medical Treatment: Treatment dependent on cause. Any underlying medical conditions should be treated.

Prognosis: Dependent on cause. Anhidrosis should improve when underlying medical condition is successfully treated. There is an increased risk of heat related illnesses such as muscle cramps, heat exhaustion and heatstroke.

Holistic Advice: Monitor physical activity levels. In warm or hot weather, wear loose fitting clothing. Try to stay cool.

Ankylosing Spondylitis

Definition: A form of arthritis that mainly affects the spine.

Possible Causes: Exact cause is unknown however there appears to be a link with a gene called GLA-B27 in many cases. This condition can run in families.

General Signs and Symptoms: Develops slowly over time and causes several parts of the lower spine to become inflamed. Over time this damage can cause parts of the spine to fuse and lose flexibility (ankylosis). Symptoms and their severity can fluctuate. The most common symptom is back pain and stiffness, which may improve with exercise and get worse with rest. Inflammation from the arthritis can affect other joints such as the hips and knees bringing symptoms of pain on moving, tenderness on examination and swelling/warmth in the area. Inflammation can also occur on the tendon or ligaments where they attach to the bone, this is called enthesitis.

Conventional Medical Treatment: There currently no cure for ankylosing spondylitis. Treatment aims to relieve symptoms and delay or prevent fusion in the spine. The main treatments are a combination of exercise, physiotherapy and medications. Physiotherapists can create tailored individual exercise programmes, give massage treatments and hydrotherapy to ease symptoms. Anti-inflammatory medication can help with inflammation. Other painkillers such as paracetamol and codeine may be prescribed. Steroid tablets and injections can also have powerful anti-inflammatory effects.

Prognosis: Lifelong treatment will be required to manage symptoms. For some people flexibility can reduce significantly over time. Joints can become damaged and osteoporosis or spinal fractures are a possibility. Those with ankylosing spondylitis are at an increased risk of cardiovascular disease. In rare occasions amyloidosis can develop where bone proteins develop in the organs.

Holistic Advice: Take regular exercise, including stretching. Maintain a healthy weight and stop smoking.

Anorexia Nervosa

Definition: An eating disorder and mental health condition characterised by not eating enough food, over exercising, or both. It can affect anyone of any age or gender.

Possible Causes: The exact cause is unknown however, there are some factors and previous life events that are thought to make it more likely including sexual abuse or a family history of eating disorders. Previous life events such as criticism around eating habits, body weight and body shape or concern around being slim, particularly if there is pressure from society or job (i.e. athletes or models). Previous mental health problems including depression and obsessive-compulsive disorder are also thought to be a risk factor.

General Signs and Symptoms: A person with anorexia will look to deliberately lose weight as well as maintain a very low body weight. Some people with anorexia will experience cycles of binging and purging. Signs of anorexia include missing meals or eating very little, lying about what has been eaten, lying about weight, taking medicine to reduce hunger, induce defecation (laxatives) or urination (diuretics). Excessive exercise and strict rituals around food are also signs of this eating disorder. Psychological symptoms experienced include an overwhelming fear of gaining weight, low confidence and self-esteem, belief that healthy weight is overweight, seeing weight loss as a positive, distorted perception of themselves, and not admitting or underestimating that the weight loss is serious. There may be other mental health problems such as depression and anxiety. Physical symptoms include cessation of menstruation (in women), unusually low BMI (body mass index), physical weakness, bloating, constipation, headaches, feeling lethargic, poor circulation in hands and feed, dry skin and hair loss. Fine, downy hair called lanugo (usually associated with newborn babies) is commonly present in adults with severe anorexia. It is important to recognise that not all people with anorexia will be underweight.

Conventional Medical Treatment: The aims of treatment are to help the person understand the causes of their eating disorder, to feel more comfortable with food and ultimately to reach a healthy weight. There are many different types of talking therapies available to help treat anorexia. These include cognitive behavioural therapy (CBT), cognitive analytic therapy (CAT), interpersonal psychotherapy (IPT) and focal psychodynamic therapy (FPT). The goal is to create a personalised treatment plan to help the person cope with their feelings, understand nutrition and starvation and make good/healthy choices with food. Medication is sometimes used in combination with talking therapies to help treat any underlying anxiety and/or depression. If the condition is severe then the person might be admitted into hospital for treatment. As a last resort, the person may be 'sectioned' for compulsory treatment under the Mental Health Act.

Prognosis: Early diagnosis and treatment often provides the best outcomes.

Prognosis Continued: Long-term effects of anorexia include osteoporosis (loss of bone density), infertility, heart issues, organ damage, weak immune system, delayed onset of puberty (in young people). It is possible for anorexia to be fatal.

Holistic Advice: Try to establish a strong support network. Engage with talking therapies on either a one to one basis or group therapy. Support groups can offer advice and information, as well as providing a forum to openly discuss feelings with those who have had similar experiences Seek an individualised treatment plan.

Appendicitis

Definition: Inflammation of the appendix.

Possible Causes: The appendix becomes filled with bacteria that produce pus, causing the appendix to swell. This can be caused by infection (e.g. a stomach infection) or an obstruction (e.g. hard piece of faeces) in the appendix that causes a bacterial infection. Sometimes the cause is unknown.

General Signs and Symptoms: Sudden onset of pain in the abdomen that shifts to the lower-right and gradually gets worse over several hours. This can be accompanied by nausea, vomiting, loss of appetite, constipation or diarrhoea, and a fever. Constant, worsening abdominal pain should be considered a medical emergency.

Conventional Medical Treatment: For mild cases antibiotics may be successful in reducing the inflammation, but in most cases the appendix will have to be surgically removed.

Prognosis: If left untreated the appendix may burst which can lead to potentially fatal consequences such as blood poisoning and peritonitis (inflammation of the abdominal lining). Removing the appendix has no detrimental effect on health and wellbeing.

Holistic Advice: It is thought that a high fibre diet may reduce the incidence of appendicitis.

<u>Asthma</u>

Definition: Intermittent narrowing of the airways, causing shortness of breath and wheezing.

Possible Causes: The bronchi become inflamed and narrow when they are irritated and mucus production increases. The muscles of the bronchi also contract making the airways narrower still. The irritation may be caused by sensitivity to certain substances, allergic reactions or other triggers, e.g. dust mites, animal fur, pollen, tobacco smoke, chemical fumes, atmospheric pollution, certain medicines, foods containing sulphites, stress, cold air and chest infections. It is thought that a combination of genetic, environmental and dietary factors may cause the condition. Risk factors include a family history of asthma, suffering from other allergic conditions (e.g. eczema), having bronchitis or being exposed to tobacco smoke as a child, being born prematurely and being born with a low birth weight.

General Signs and Symptoms: Difficulty breathing, breathlessness, wheezing, coughing and a tight chest. The severity of asthma attacks vary enormously from mild to life threatening. Symptoms such as an increase in pulse rate, more wheezing, and a feeling of agitation or restlessness, can indicate that the attack is worsening. In a severe attack, breathing may become very difficult, causing the lips and finger nails to turn blue, the nostrils to flare and pulse race. A severe attack should be treated as a medical emergency.

Conventional Medical Treatment: The aim is to eliminate symptoms and reduce the severity and frequency of future attacks. Medicines are usually administered using an inhaler. Bronchodilators are used to help alleviate the symptoms, and corticosteroids can be given to help prevent another attack. Lifestyle changes and diet play an important role.

Prognosis: The narrowing of the airways is usually reversible, either occurring naturally or with the use of medicines. However, in some chronic cases the inflammation may lead to an irreversible obstruction of the airways. Asthma can lead to serious respiratory complications and can be fatal.

Holistic Advice: Stop smoking. Maintain a healthy weight, keep to a healthy diet and exercise regularly. Yoga and gentle exercise can help keep the whole body in balance, thus helping it to cope with asthma and its associated anxiety. Practitioners should be fully trained to deal with asthmatic attacks before treating patients with asthma. During an attack, always remain calm and reassure the person. Seek medical advice if the condition worsens or persists.

Atherosclerosis

Definition: A progressive condition in which the medium and large arteries become clogged by cholesterol and fatty substances. It is a type of arteriosclerosis and can attribute to cardiovascular diseases such as heart attacks, strokes, coronary heart disease and peripheral artery disease.

Possible Causes: Arteries naturally begin to harden and narrow with age but the process can be accelerated by high fat diets and high "bad" cholesterol (low density lipoprotein) levels. The cholesterol sticks to the wall of the arteries and the fatty deposits (atheroma) build up over time. Platelets may worsen the condition by collecting on the fatty deposits forming blood clots. Risk factors include smoking, lack of exercise, hypertension, being overweight, diabetes, high alcohol intake, family history, ethnicity and air pollution.

General Signs and Symptoms: Symptoms do not usually arise until the blood flow becomes restricted or blocked and then the symptoms depend on the location of the arteries affected. For example, if the atherosclerosis is in the arteries of the legs, causing peripheral artery disease, cramping pains and numbness will be felt in the lower limbs. This pain is called intermittent claudication. Angina is brought on by atherosclerosis of the coronary arteries and the narrowing of these arteries can lead to a heart attack. Blood clots can form as a result of atherosclerosis and cause heart attacks (if in the coronary arteries) and stokes (if blood supply to the brain is restricted). Atherosclerosis can also weaken the artery walls causing bulges called aneurysms. If the aneurysm ruptures the blood loss can prove fatal.

Conventional Medical Treatment: The treatment focuses on preventing the condition from getting worse and triggering cardiovascular disease. Drugs can be used to lessen the risk factors by lowering cholesterol levels (e.g. statins), lowering blood pressure (e.g. ACE inhibitors), and preventing blood clots (e.g. anti-platelets and aspirin). Surgery may be possible to widen the affected artery or bypass the restriction.

Prognosis: Lifestyle changes and medication can slow the progress. Left untreated the outlook is poor and it is a major cause of a heart attack, stroke and poor peripheral circulation.

Holistic Advice: Lifestyle changes are very important to prevent the condition or to prevent the condition from worsening. Stop smoking and lose any excess weight. Take regular exercise and reduce stress levels. Maintain a healthy low fat, high fibre diet.

Athlete's Foot

Definition: Fungal disease of the skin on the feet, commonly between the toes. Also known as tinea pedis.

Possible Causes: Fungal infection caused by the fungus dermatophyte, yeasts and moulds, often picked up in warm places with humid environments such as swimming pools and changing rooms. Can also be caused by the constant sweating of the feet which causes the bacteria on the feet to multiply and infect the skin. It is contagious and so care must be taken to avoid direct or indirect contact.

General Signs and Symptoms: In the area of the infection the skin tends to be inflamed, moist, flaky, itchy and painful. Sometimes it has small blisters or a rash. In severe cases, toenails can be affected and may crumble and separate from the nail bed.

Conventional Medical Treatment: Antifungal creams, sprays and liquids applied topically will usually quickly clear up the infection. In severe cases, a GP may prescribe oral antifungal drugs.

Prognosis: If treated effectively, the infection will usually clear up in a few days or weeks. Untreated it can last for several month, even years.

Holistic Advice: Wash feet regularly, ensuring they are dried properly – particularly between the toes. Foot powder preparations can be bought without prescription to help the feet dry out. Change socks everyday! Cotton socks are best. Avoid sharing towels to help prevent any infection from spreading.

Atony

Definition: When a muscle loses its strength.

Possible Causes: Dependent on the area affected. Can be due to trauma, neurological or hormonal reasons. Examples of where atony can occur include atonic seizure (neurological but exact cause is unknown), uterine atony (hormonal and/or trauma of childbirth) and atonic colon (cause most often unknown, rarely Hirschsprung's Disease).

General Signs and Symptoms: Dependent on the area affected. In an atonic seizure (also known as a drop attack), all the muscles will suddenly go limp and the person will often fall to the floor. Other symptoms such as dropping eyelids, head nods and jerking may be experienced. Uterine atony is characterised by excessively bleeding post-partum, decreased heart rate, pain and a non-contracted uterus. The main symptom of atonic colon is constipation. Stomach pain, bloating, nausea, vomiting and fever may also be experienced.

Conventional Medical Treatment: Dependent on the underlying cause and area affected.

Prognosis: Dependent on the underlying cause. Uterine atony is a common cause of post-partum haemorrhage and can be life threating.

Holistic Advice: Specific diets and getting enough sleep can help with atonic seizure. High fibre diets may be beneficial for some instances of atonic colon.

Atrophy

Definition: The wasting or loss of muscle tissue.

Possible Causes: Muscle atrophy can occur due to a number of reasons. Lack of physical activity for a long period of time (e.g. being bedridden due to illness or injury), natural ageing, malnutrition, stoke, spinal cord injury and long term steroid therapy. Conditions such as muscular dystrophy, multiple sclerosis, arthritis, polio and neuropathy can all cause reduced mobility and contribute to muscular atrophy.

General Signs and Symptoms: The muscles in one of the arms or legs may appear noticeably smaller. This can be coupled with marked weakness in that limb.

Conventional Medical Treatment: Dependent on cause and severity of atrophy. Underlying medication conditions should be treated as quickly as possible. Exercise and physical therapy can be used to slowly build muscle and strength in the area over time. If malnutrition is the cause then a personalised nutrition programme might be recommended.

Prognosis: Can be reversed through regular exercise, proper nutrition and successfully treating any underlying health conditions.

Holistic Advice: Eat a healthy balanced diet and exercise regularly.

Back Pain

Definition: Pain anywhere along the spine.

Possible Causes: Back pain can be non-specific (no identifiable cause) or due to a minor injury such as a sprain or strain (mechanical). Lower back pain (lumbago) is the most common. Medical conditions such as slipped disc(s), sciatica, ankylosing spondylitis and spondylolisthesis can all cause back pain and will have specific treatment plans. Very rarely, back pain can be caused by a broken bone in the spine, infection, cancer and cauda equine syndrome. Risk factors for developing back pain are poor posture, long periods of inactivity and being overweight.

General Signs and Symptoms: Pain anywhere along the spine from the neck to the hips. The pain can range from a dull ache to a shooting or stabbing pain. Specific movements such as bending, twisting or lifting may make the pain worse.

Conventional Medical Treatment: Symptoms are often mild and require no formal treatment. Keeping active, performing stretches for the back and taking anti-inflammatory painkillers will usually help the episode to pass. Using hot or cold packs can help relieve symptoms. If pain and symptoms cannot be managed at home referral to a physiotherapist may be required. Surgery is only recommended if there is a medical condition causing the back pain and other treatments have not worked.

Prognosis: Symptoms will usually resolve on their own after a few weeks.

Holistic Advice: Maintain a healthy weight and take regular exercise. Avoid sitting for long periods of time.

Bell's Palsy

Definition: Weakness or paralysis of the muscles on one side of the face. The eyelid may also be affected.

Possible Causes: Damage to the facial nerve as a result of inflammation, compression or a direct wound. Victims of apoplexy (stroke) may also show symptoms of Bell's palsy. Facial palsy, of which Bell's palsy is one type, may be associated with shingles (a viral infection) and Lyme disease (a bacterial infection carried by ticks).

General Signs and Symptoms: Weakness or paralysis on one side of the face, difficulty in closing the eye, and the drooping of one side of mouth which causes drooling and speech impairment. The eye may become dry, due to the eyelid being unable to close. Pain may be experienced underneath the ear and the sense of taste may be affected. The symptoms tend to develop quickly.

Conventional Medical Treatment: Steroids to reduce the inflammation. The eye on the affected side must also be cared for to ensure it is kept clean and moist. Eye drops and ointments are commonly prescribed for this.

Prognosis: Most show an improvement within 3 weeks and 85% make a full recovery within 9 months. Long lasting nerve damage is possible but rare.

Holistic Advice: Gentle massage concentrating on the back of the head and neck may help. Consult a qualified massage practitioner. Acupressure or acupuncture may be useful in the initial stages.

Benign Prostatic Enlargement

Definition: Enlarged prostate not usually a serious threat to health.

Possible Causes: Exact cause is unknown. Common in men aged over 50 and thought to be linked to hormonal changes.

General Signs and Symptoms: The enlarged prostate can place pressure on the bladder and urethra causing difficulty in passing urine, increased frequency of urination, urinary incontinence and difficulty fully emptying the bladder.

Conventional Medical Treatment: Mild symptoms often do not require immediate treatment but regular check-ups will be advised. If lifestyle changes do not help or are unsuitable, medicines to relax the prostate, shrink the prostrate, increase urine production and slow down urine production may be prescribed. If trouble with urination persists, a catheter may be inserted to drain the bladder. If other treatments have not worked, there are a number of surgical procedures to remove part or all of the prostate or increase the size of the bladder.

Prognosis: Complications can include urinary tract infections (UTI) and acute urinary retention (sudden inability to pass urine). No additional risk of prostate cancer.

Holistic Advice: Lifestyle changes such as consuming less alcohol, caffeine, fizzy drinks and artificial sweeteners. Take regular exercise. See a GP if any of the above symptoms are experienced, even if mild.

Bipolar Disorder

Definition: A mental health condition that affects a person's mood causing episodes of depression and mania. Formerly known as manic depression.

Possible Causes: Exact cause is unknown and is thought to develop via a complex mix of social, physical and environmental factors. There is evidence to suggest that chemical imbalances in the brain, specifically neurotransmitters, can cause symptoms of bipolar disorder to develop. Certain stressful situations such as a physical illness, a relationship breaking down, abuse (physical, sexual or emotional) and the death of a loved one can trigger symptoms of bipolar disorder. Those with a family member with bipolar disorder have an increased risk of developing it.

General Signs and Symptoms: Episodes of depression (low mood) and mania (high mood), often lasting weeks or months at a time. Patterns of episodes can vary and sometimes there will be periods of 'normal' mood. Symptoms will be dependent on the mood that is being experienced. Episodes of depression include feeling sad/hopeless, difficulty concentrating, feelings of emptiness, guilt and despair. Additionally, a lack of appetite, difficulty sleeping and suicidal thoughts can be experienced. Manic episodes are characterised by feeling happy, full of energy, talking quickly, not eating and being easily distracted. Sometimes there may be illogical thinking and some may make decisions that have grave consequences such as spending large quantities of money.

Conventional Medical Treatment: Treatment aims to reduce the severity and number of episodes. Lithium, anticonvulsant and antipsychotic medicines can all be used to help stabilise mood swings. A mental health professional can help individuals learn to recognise the warning signs of an approaching episode. Cognitive behaviour therapy (CBT) can be useful for depression.

Prognosis: Effective treatment can reduce the length of episodes. Care should be taken if trying to become pregnant whilst on medication for bipolar disorder. Some treatments can increase the risk of developing diabetes.

Holistic Advice: Eat a healthy balanced diet and exercise regularly. Avoid drugs and alcohol. Avoid stressful situations.

Bladder Stones

Definition: Small deposits of minerals that form in the bladder.

Possible Causes: If urine remains in the bladder for too long, waste products in the urine can crystallize and form stones. Bladder stones are therefore often caused by conditions in which the ability of the bladder to fully empty is compromised, e.g. recurrent bladder infections, prostatitis, and neurological problems that affect bladder control. Other risk factors include a diet high in fat, sugar or salt, prolonged dehydration, metabolic conditions such as gout (due to the increased levels of waste products in the urine), and vitamin A or B deficiency.

General Signs and Symptoms: Some bladder stones can be passed from the bladder unnoticed. Usually, however, symptoms are experienced because the stones can irritate the wall of the bladder or block the flow of urine. Symptoms include pain when urinating, blood in the urine, lower abdominal pain, difficulty beginning to urinate, stop-start urination, the need to urinate frequently and the need to urinate in the night. Bladder stones are more common in men than women, and are more common over the age of 45.

Conventional Medical Treatment: Small stones may be flushed out by drinking more water. It may be possible to break larger stones down using lithotripsy, which involves sending high-energy shock waves through the stone to break it up so the pieces can then be flushed out. Alternatively, stones can be surgically removed.

Prognosis: Treatment to remove the stones is usually successful, but if the underlying cause remains they may recur.

Holistic Advice: Drink plenty of water. Eat a low fat, high fibre diet with plenty of fresh fruit and vegetables. Limit sugar and salt intake.

Blisters

Definition: Small pockets of clear fluid (serum) under the upper layers of skin.

Possible Causes: Blisters form to protect an area of damaged skin and are most commonly caused by friction, burns (e.g. chemical, scalds and UV radiation) and allergic reactions. Conditions such a chickenpox, cold sores, genital herpes, bullous impetigo, scabies and hand, foot and mouth disease can all cause blisters.

General Signs and Symptoms: Characterised by a raised 'bubble' of skin with clear fluid inside. Blisters can be filled with blood and be red in colour if the underlying blood vessels have been damaged too. Blood blisters are often more painful than normal blisters. Infected blisters will be filled with green or yellow pus and the surrounding skin may be red and warm to touch.

Conventional Medical Treatment: Small blisters caused by injury to the skin will not require any treatment and can be covered with a soft plaster. To prevent infection and promote healing in bigger blisters, hydrocolloid dressings can be worn. Large or very painful blisters can be lanced with a sterilised needle or scalpel by a doctor or trained professional. Antibiotics will be prescribed for infection. Underlying conditions that cause blisters should be treated.

Prognosis: The large majority of blisters will resolve by themselves. If left untreated infected blisters can cause cellulitis and sepsis.

Holistic Advice: Do not burst the blister. If the blister bursts itself, do not remove the skin or pick at the edges and wash hands properly before touching it. Wear comfortable well-fitting shoes and clean socks to help prevent blisters on the feet. Wear protective gloves when handling chemicals. Wear high factor sun cream to prevent sunburn.

Boils

Definition: A red, painful, pus-filled swelling of the skin. A cluster of boils is referred to as a carbuncle.

Possible Causes: Bacterial infection (usually Staphylococcus aureus) of the hair follicle or sebaceous gland. As the infection spreads pus collects in the surrounding tissues. Most common in those with a low resistance to infection such as diabetics or those with HIV. Carbuncles are less common and mostly affect middle-aged men.

General Signs and Symptoms: Small, red, tender lump that feels warm to the touch and throbs. The tissues around the boil swell as pus accumulates. Eventually the boil forms a yellow or white head. Boils are commonly located on the neck or face, in moist areas of the body such as the armpits, and in areas subjected to friction from clothing. They are most common in teenagers and young adults. Boils can collect together to form carbuncles. These clusters fill with pus and can weep, ooze or even rupture. Carbuncles can cause fever and swelling of nearby lymph nodes depending on the location.

Conventional Medical Treatment: Antibiotics may be needed if the infection looks to be spreading to the deeper layers of the skin. Doctors may drain the pus if necessary. Large boils or carbuncles may need to be lanced. Painkillers may be required to treat the pain.

Prognosis: Most heal without treatment within a couple of weeks. They may burst and release the pus or gradually subside. Recurrent boils may be indicative of an underlying medical condition. Secondary infections, most commonly cellulitis, are a risk if the infection spreads. Deep carbuncles could cause scarring. In rare cases, carbuncles can cause sepsis.

Holistic Advice: Do not squeeze the boil. The healing process may be improved by applying a cloth, made hot by soaking in warm water, to the boil for 10 minutes, 3-4 times a day. Wash your hands after touching the boil or carbuncle and wash any clothes, bedding or towels that have had contact with the boil/carbuncle. Try to improve the immune system.

Bone Cancer

Definition: Cancer that begins in the bone(s). The main types include osteosarcoma, Ewing sarcoma and chondrosarcoma.

Possible Causes: Exact cause is often unknown and can develop in any bone though the long bones of the arm and legs are most common. Risk factors for developing bone cancers include previous radiotherapy treatment, having other bone conditions such as Paget's disease, genetic conditions such as Li-Fraumeni syndrome and previous history of other cancers in childhood such as retinoblastoma.

General Signs and Symptoms: Dependent on which bone(s) are affected. Bone pain is the most common symptom experienced. This usually starts with tenderness and progresses to persistent ache that is present even at rest. In some cases, swelling and inflammation may be present on the affected bone. If this is close to a joint, the inflammation can make the joint hard to use properly. The affect bone may become weak due the cancer and fracture easily. Less commonly fever, sweating and unexplained weight loss may occur.

Conventional Medical Treatment: Dependent on the type and stage. Surgery is often recommended to remove the bone affected by the cancer. This may be limb sparing (removing a section of the affected bone and tissue) or amputation. Chemotherapy and radiotherapy can be used in combination with surgery. Medication can be used for osteosarcoma to encourage the immune system to produce cancer killing cells.

Prognosis: Dependent on type, stage and grade (how likely it is to spread further). Most stage 1 and stage 2 bone cancers have a good chance of being cured through treatment. Stage 3 bone cancers are more difficult and the main aim will be to slow the spread of the cancer.

Holistic Advice: Gentle physical exercise and a healthy balanced diet can help prepare the body for treatment. Support groups can be of use.

Brain Aneurysm

Definition: An outward bulge in the blood vessel wall, usually where it branches. The medical term is an intracranial or cerebral aneurysm.

Possible Causes: Weakness in the blood vessel walls in the brain. The exact cause of an aneurysm is often unclear but there are several factors that increase the risk of one developing including smoking, high blood pressure, family history of brain aneurysm, age (risk increases as you get older), being female and cocaine abuse. Some conditions also increase risk of developing aneurysm such as congenital heart disease, autosomal dominant polycystic kidney disease, Ehler-Danlos syndrome and Marfan syndrome. In very rare cases, people who have experienced severe head trauma can develop a brain aneurysm.

General Signs and Symptoms: Most brain aneurysms only show symptoms upon rupture (bursting). A ruptured brain aneurysm leads to a condition called subarachnoid haemorrhage and most commonly presents as a sudden, extremely intense headache, unlike anything experienced before. Other symptoms may include nausea, vomiting, neck pain, light sensitivity, confusion, blurred vision, seizures, confusion and weakness on one side of the body. Occasionally a formed brain aneurysm will cause vision loss, pain around the eye, numbness or weakness on one side of the face, headache, speech difficulties, loss of concentration and balance.

Conventional Medical Treatment: If still intact, treatment will depend on the risk of the aneurysm rupturing which can be affected by age, size of the aneurysm, location, family history and underlying health conditions such as high blood pressure. Surgery, such as a neurosurgical clipping or endovascular coiling can be used as a preventative measure. If the aneurysm has ruptured, it is a medical emergency. Medication will be used to attempt to reduce the risk of the brains blood supply being severely compromised. Then, one of the above coiling or clipping surgeries will be performed.

Prognosis: If the assessed risks are low there is only a small chance the aneurysm rupturing. Many people will not know that they have a brain aneurysm as there are often no symptoms. If the aneurysm ruptures, there is a very high chance of death, even with emergency surgery. Those who survive are often left with severe brain damage and disability.

Holistic Advice: Stop smoking. Maintain normal blood pressure by eating a healthy balanced diet, maintaining a healthy weight and exercising regularly. Reduce alcohol and caffeine intake.

Brain Tumour

Definition: Cancerous (malignant) or non-cancerous (benign) tumour found in the brain.

Possible Causes: Exact cause is often unknown. The risk of developing a brain tumour increases with age and there are certain rare genetic conditions that can also contribute. Lifestyle factors such as being overweight or obese can increase the risk of brain tumour. In rare cases, brain tumours can be caused by previous radiotherapy treatments. Family history of the disease is also a risk factor.

General Signs and Symptoms: Dependent on the area where the tumour has developed. Common symptoms are headaches, seizures, nausea, vomiting, memory issues, changes in personality, weakness and vison or speech problems.

Conventional Medical Treatment: Dependent on the location, type, size and grade of the tumour. Low grade tumours are usually benign and slow growing whereas high grade tumours are usually cancerous and fast growing. Surgery is the most common treatment and will attempt to remove as much of the tumour as possible. Chemotherapy and radiotherapy can be used to destroy the tumour cells. Medication can be used to help control seizures, reduce brain swelling and control pain.

Prognosis: Dependent on the location, type, size and grade of the tumour. After treatment there may be lasting problems such as seizures, mobility issues and speech problems. Treatment can also cause cataracts, epilepsy and cognitive problems. It is common for brain tumours to reoccur.

Holistic Advice: Take regular gentle exercise and eat a healthy balanced diet. Stop smoking and avoid contact sports.

Breast Cancer

Definition: Cancer of the breast tissue. Usually described as non-invasive (in the ducts of the breast) or invasive (spread through the ducts into the breast tissue).

Possible Causes: Exact causes are unknown however, risk factors include; age (risk increases over 50), family history of breast/ovarian cancer, previous diagnosis, previous benign breast lump, being overweight or obese and alcohol consumption. In men, genetics/family history and conditions increasing levels of oestrogen in the body such as obesity and cirrhosis are thought to increase risk.

General Signs and Symptoms: Any change in the appearance of the breast including; a new lump in either breast, change in size or shape of either breast, a rash on or discharge from the nipples, lump or swelling in the armpits and dimpling of the skin on either breast. In men, cancerous breast lumps usually only occur in one breast, under/around the nipple. In both women and men, most lumps are benign, however they should always been checked by a doctor.

Conventional Medical Treatment: Often a combination of treatments and dependent on how early the cancer is diagnosed. The main treatments are; surgery (where the breast is conserved or removed in a mastectomy), radiotherapy and chemotherapy. Hormone therapy may be used in combination with other treatments if the breast cancer is sensitive to hormones. Targeted therapy can be used to change the way cells work to reduce or stop the growth and spread of the cancer.

Prognosis: There is a good chance of successful recovery if the cancer is caught early in both women and men. Long-terms complications of treatment is rare. Sometimes pain/stiffness can occur post-operation. Chemotherapy can bring about early menopause.

Holistic Advice: Check breasts regularly for any changes. If aged between 50 – 70 ensure you attend a screening every three years. Maintain a healthy diet and weight, take regular exercise and limit the intake of alcohol. Complementary therapies are encouraged to promote physical and emotional well-being in particular breathing exercises, massage, aromatherapy, reflexology and acupuncture.

Breast Lump

Definition: A mass or swelling that can be felt in the breast tissue.

Possible Causes: Generalised lumpiness is often associated with hormonal changes at puberty, pregnancy and menstruation due to the oversensitivity of the breast tissue to female sex hormones. Mastitis (inflammation of the breast tissue) can cause breast lumps. One of the most common causes of breast lumps in pre-menopausal women is fibroadenosis. This is caused by the formation of excessive fibrous connective tissue that causes breast pain, breast enlargement and general lumpiness of the breast. One type of non-malignant breast tumour is fibroadenoma. These tumours (solid masses) can be felt as hard rubbery lumps and may be caused by an overgrowth of fibrous and glandular tissue. Fibroadenoma is most common in women in their 20s. Breast cysts (fluid filled sac in the breast tissue) can be felt as lumps too. Occasionally the breast lump may be due to an infection that has caused the development of an abscess. Lumps may also be caused by injury and fatty growths. A breast lump can also be symptomatic of breast cancer, although 9 out of 10 breast lumps are benign.

General Signs and Symptoms: Generalised lumpiness in the breast tissue or a separate, individual lump felt either deep in the breast tissue or just under the skin. There may be breast pain. The skin may dimple and the lump may cause inversion of the nipple and a bloody nipple discharge. Specific signs and symptoms vary according to the cause.

Conventional Medical Treatment: Generalised lumpiness tends to decrease after the menopause. Drugs can be given to help reduce breast pain. Small fibroadenomas do not usually need treatment and tend to become smaller or disappear within a couple of years. Larger fibroadenomas may need to be removed surgically or by laser. Breast cysts and abscesses can be drained. A variety of treatments is available for breast cancer, including lumpectomy, mastectomy, radiotherapy, chemotherapy and other drug treatments such as tamoxifen.

Prognosis: Benign breast lumps are harmless and most do not need treatment. Lumps due to breast cancer are serious. Early diagnosis significantly affects the outcome. If diagnosed before the cancer has spread to other body organs then the treatment is more likely to be successful.

Holistic Advice: Check the breasts regularly for any lumps. Any changes in the breast should be reported to a Doctor. Reduce caffeine intake and cut down on fatty foods. Wear a good supporting bra.

Bromhidrosis

Definition: Unpleasant or offensive body odour. Also knowns as osmidrosis.

Possible Causes: Body odour occurs when bacteria on the surface of the skin break down sweat, sebum and keratin. Body odour is normal but can become offensive or unpleasant through bad hygiene practices, infection and skin disorders. The smell of body odour can be affected by certain foods such as garlic, onion, alcohol and asparagus.

General Signs and Symptoms: Unpleasant of offensive body odour that the person is often unaware of.

Conventional Medical Treatment: Treatment should aim to target any underlying causes such as infection. Hair removal and exfoliation can help reduce unpleasant odours.

Prognosis: Treating the underlying cause can stop bromhidrosis completely. It may not be possible to completely supress it and there can be significant impacts on mental health including increased anxiety and lowered self-esteem.

Holistic Advice: Practice good personal hygiene and wash clothes regularly.

Bronchiolitis

Definition: A lower respiratory tract infection in the bronchioles affecting babies and children under 2.

Possible Causes: Almost always caused by the respiratory syncytial virus (RSV), the bronchioles become inflamed which reduces the amount of air able to enter the lungs. Spread directly through close contact with people via droplets expelled into the air via coughs and sneezes. Most commonly found in babies between 3 – 6 months of age.

General Signs and Symptoms: General symptoms are very similar to the common cold i.e. blocking/runny nose (non-allergic rhinitis), sneezing and coughing. Fever, difficulty feeding and wheezing will usually develop over the next few days. In severe cases breathing difficulties may develop.

Conventional Medical Treatment: The large majority of cases will not need any medical intervention and can be treated at home - in the same way that the common cold would be. Some children may need to be admitted to hospital if they have breathing difficulties. Paracetamol or ibuprofen can be used for fever.

Prognosis: A full recovery is expected within 2 weeks.

Holistic Advice: Provide the child with plenty of fluids, keep them warm and encourage rest. Practice good hand hygiene (for parent and child) and wipe surfaces regularly. Keep new born babies away from other people who have a cold or flu. Do not smoke around your child.

Bronchitis

Definition: Inflammation of the mucous membrane within the bronchial tubes.

Possible Causes: Acute bronchitis is caused by a bacterial or, more commonly, a viral infection, often developing after a cold, sore throat or flu. Smokers, those with other pulmonary (lung) diseases, and those exposed to substances that can irritate the lungs are at greater risk. In such cases the condition may become chronic.

General Signs and Symptoms: The symptoms will vary according to the severity of the attack and the extent of the inflammation. At first the symptoms of acute bronchitis can be similar to those of a common cold (e.g. sore throat, headache, blocked nose, aches and pains and a slight fever). The main symptom is a cough that may remain long after the other symptoms have gone. The cough is usually short, dry and painful at first, with fast wheezes of respiration. The chest becomes painful and tight and, as the disease progresses, the cough may become productive.

Conventional Medical Treatment: Painkillers (such as paracetamol) can be used to reduce any temperature and help with the aches. Should a secondary infection arise (usually indicated by coughing up discoloured sputum), antibiotics may be prescribed. Antibiotics are not commonly prescribed for acute bronchitis because it is usually caused by a viral infection and so they would serve no purpose.

Prognosis: Acute bronchitis is usually mild and clears up by itself. There is no cure for chronic bronchitis but lifestyle changes may help.

Holistic Advice: During an attack drink plenty of water and rest. Give up smoking and avoid smoky areas. Take advice on breathing exercises.

Bulimia Nervosa

Definition: An eating disorder and mental health condition characterised by binge eating and purging. It can affect anyone of any age or gender but typically develops during adolescence or early adulthood.

Possible Causes: The exact cause is unknown however, there are some factors and previous life events that are thought to make it more likely including sexual abuse or a family history of eating disorders. Previous life events such as criticism around eating habits, body weight and body shape or concern around being slim, particularly if there is pressure from society or job (i.e. athletes or models). Previous mental health problems including depression, obsessive-compulsive disorder and anxiety are also thought to be a risk factor.

General Signs and Symptoms: The main sign of bulimia is binge/purge cycles. These are characterised by eating large amounts of food over short time period and then purging the body of that food by inducing vomiting, defecation (using laxatives) or excessively exercising (or a combination of all three). Psychological symptoms include spending a lot of time thinking about food, low confidence, fear of putting on weight, feelings of guilt, avoiding social activities that involve food, low mood, anxiety and feeling critical of one's appearance. Physical symptoms such as lethargy, constipation, weight fluctuation, sore throat, tooth decay, bloating and self-harm can also be experienced.

Conventional Medical Treatment: Therapy is often recommended for people with bulimia. A personalised self-help programme is usually the initial treatment that will help the person monitor their eating habits, make meal plans, identify the underlying cause of the bulimia and learn about what triggers their binge/purge cycle. Cognitive behavioural therapy (CBT) specifically for bulimia can also be used. Medication is sometimes used in combination with self-help or CBT to help treat any underlying anxiety and/or depression. If the condition is severe then the person might be admitted into hospital for treatment

Prognosis: Treatment may take time but a full recovery is possible. Long-term effects of bulimia include permanent damage to the teeth, damage to the throat and vocal cords, damage to the digestive tract, heart problems and kidney damage. It is possible for bulimia to be fatal.

Holistic Advice: Whilst recovering drink plenty of water to keep hydrated. Try not to drink or eat very acidic foods during a binge and after purging. Rinse the mouth the non-acidic mouthwash and avoid brushing the teeth immediately after vomiting.

Bunions

Definition: A bony swelling at the base of the big toe. Called hallux valgus.

Possible Causes: Exact cause is not known but bunions may be familial. Badly fitting shoes may also be a contributing factor. They can be caused or worsened by arthritis.

General Signs and Symptoms: Big toe bends towards the middle of the foot and the second toe creating a swollen, red, bony lump on the medial edge of the foot where the first and second metatarsals are pushed apart. The skin over the bump can become thick, rough and may break. There may be pain on walking, particularly if wearing tight footwear or high heels. Bunions are more common in women than men (probably because of the high-heeled shoes!).

Conventional Medical Treatment: Treatment is only necessary if the bunion is causing pain, which may be controlled simply by wearing flat, wide shoes. Painkillers can be taken, and bunion pads and ice packs may be effective. However, bunions will only worsen over time and the only cure for them is corrective surgery.

Prognosis: Surgery is generally successful in straightening the joint and relieving the pain. However, as with all surgery, there is the chance that complications will arise. Bunion surgery can cause stiffness in the joint, pain under the ball of the foot, nerve damage and infection. There is also no guarantee that the bunion will not reform.

Holistic Advice: Wear shoes that fit – preferably wide enough to allow the toes space to move.

Burns and Scalds

Definition: Damage to the skin by heat. Burns are caused by dry heat such as fire and scalds are caused by wet heat such as boiling water.

Possible Causes: Burns can be caused by a variety of things such as fire, hot drinks, an iron, kettle or cooker/stove. Faulty electrical items can also cause burns as well as specific types of chemicals. Exposure to UV radiation from the sun without appropriate sun protection can cause sunburn.

General Signs and Symptoms: Characterised by redness, peeling skin, blisters swelling or white/charred skin. Burns can often be very painful but in some instances they may be painless. There are 4 main types of burn which have difference appearances and symptoms. Superficial epidermal burns are where the outer layer of skin (epidermis) is damaged. There will be redness, slight swelling and pain but no blisters. Superficial dermal burn is where the outer layer (epidermis) and part of the dermis (middle layer) is damaged. The skin will be pale pink, painful and potentially some small blisters. Deep dermal/partial thickness burns are where the outer layer (epidermis) and dermis are damaged. The skin will be red, blotchy, swollen and blistered. It can be very painful or completely painless. Full thickness burns are the most severe where all three layers (epidermis, dermis and subcutaneous) are damaged. The skin will be burnt away and the tissue underneath will appear pale or blackened.

Conventional Medical Treatment: Dependent on the cause and severity. Minor burns should be possible to treat at home. In all cases, the person should be removed from the heat source and the burn should be cooled under cool/lukewarm water for twenty minutes. Remove clothing/jewellery close to the affected area but do not remove anything stuck to skin. To protect the area, cover it with cling film (if possible). Serious burns such as large burns (bigger than hand sized), burns that cause charred skin, burns that blister or chemical/electrical burns should be referred to A&E where they will be cleaned and covered. In some cases surgery will be required to replace the burnt skin with health tissue from elsewhere on the body. This is called a skin graft.

Prognosis: Mild burns that affect the outer layer of the skin (superficial epidermal burns) should heal quickly with no scarring. Superficial dermal burns normally heal over 2 weeks and leave minimal scaring. More severe and deeper burns can take a very long time to heal and often leave visible scarring. Burns are susceptible to infection and there is a risk of sepsis or toxic shock syndrome.

Holistic Advice: Do not burst any blisters that form and keep the burn as clean as possible. If the inside of the mouth is scalded avoid hot drinks, smoking and spicy food until it has healed.

Bursitis

Definition: Inflammation of a bursa. Bursae are fluid-filled sacs that act as cushions between surfaces that rub together such as bones, muscles, joints and tendons, reducing friction between them.

Possible Causes: Bursae can become inflamed by injury most often as a result of repetitive action. Occasionally the inflammation may be due to infection, but this only tends to occur in those with a weakened immune system. Bursitis can also be symptomatic of joint conditions such as rheumatoid arthritis and gout. Risk factors include any activity that involves repetitive movement (e.g. joggers' ankles are at risk, as are the knees of those who regularly kneel, such as gardeners and carpet fitters) and factors that weaken the immune system, such as diabetes, HIV/AIDS, cancer treatments and heavy alcohol consumption.

General Signs and Symptoms: Pain and swelling in the affected area. This is commonly a joint such as the shoulder (deltoid bursitis), elbow, knee (called housemaid's knee), ankle, heel (Achilles bursitis) and hip, but may also occur on the thighs (through stretching) and buttocks (from sitting on hard surfaces). Joints may become difficult to move due to the inflammation.

Conventional Medical Treatment: Symptoms are often mild and require no treatment. Rest and taking painkillers (such as ibuprofen) will usually help the episode to pass. Protecting the area from further damage and using ice packs and compression can help. Elevating the affected area (if possible) may also help the inflammation.

Prognosis: Symptoms usually pass in a couple of weeks.

Holistic Advice: Protect joints that are at risk (e.g. use knee pads if often kneeling). Take regular breaks from repetitive actions and warm up adequately before exercise. Boost the immune system. Maintaining muscle strength and tone will help protect joints.

Cancer

Definition: Term used to describe malignant disease. There are many types of cancer, usually named after the area of the body affected – e.g. breast cancer, lung cancer, prostate cancer, pancreatic cancer. The disease may then spread through the blood and lymphatic systems. There are many different terms used to describe the type of cancer such as malignant tumours (as solid mass of cells), carcinoma (malignant epithelial tumour), sarcoma (malignant tumour of the connective tissue), malignant melanoma (cancer affecting the pigment cells in the skin that can spread to other parts of the body), lymphoma (cancer of the lymphatic system), and leukaemia (cancer of bone marrow in which the white blood cells multiply uncontrollably).

Possible Causes: A cell may become cancerous when certain genes that control vital processes such as cell division become damaged. These faulty genes may be inherited or caused by carcinogens (cancer-causing agents) such as tobacco smoke and sunlight. Most cancers appear to be triggered by several factors, inherited and environmental. Key environmental factors also include diet, environmental pollution, alcohol, viral infections, age and hormonal influences. There may be psychological factors involved too. Depression, grief and severe mental stresses may affect vulnerability.

General Signs and Symptoms: The body's cells begin to grow and reproduce in an uncontrollable way. These cancer cells invade healthy tissue and destroy it. The majority of cancers produce a solid tumour in a specific part of the body. The signs and symptoms vary according to the location of the tumour e.g. cancer of the stomach may cause dyspepsia; cancer of the bowel may produce diarrhoea or constipation; lymphoma may cause persistent and painless swellings in the neck, armpits, or groin caused by enlarged lymph glands. Skin cancers may be seen as hard swellings on the skin's surface that may break down and ulcerate.

Conventional Medical Treatment: The treatment is determined by the type of cancer and its severity.

Prognosis: Varies from type to type. Early diagnosis is very important.

Holistic Advice: Eating a healthy diet, taking regular exercise and not smoking may all contribute to preventing cancer.

Candida

Definition: The name for a group of yeasts that cause infection, known as candidiasis. When affecting the mouth or genitals it is referred to as thrush.

Possible Causes: The most common Candida to cause candidiasis is Candida albicans. Candida needs a living host to survive and often lives harmlessly in and on the human body. If the immune system of the host is lowered it can cause infection in the mouth, anus, genitals, skin, nails and very rarely progress to systemic infection. Candidasis is more likely in infancy or old age with conditions such as diabetes, Cushing syndrome, psoriasis and HIV more likely to develop infection. Long term antibiotic use and immunosuppressive medications can also cause candidiasis to occur.

General Signs and Symptoms: Dependent on the area infected.

Conventional Medical Treatment: Dependent on the area infected. Most commonly anti-fungal medications are taken orally or topically applied to the area that is affected.

Prognosis: Treatment is usually effective but the infection can recur.

Holistic Advice: Take steps to boost the immune system.

Cardiac Arrhythmia

Definition: An abnormality in the normal rhythm of the heart. There are many types including atrial fibrillation (irregular and fast), ventricular fibrillation (irregular and fast), supraventricular tachycardia (episodes of abnormally fast at rest), bradycardia (abnormally slow) and heart block (abnormally slow). We will focus on tachycardia and bradycardia here.

Possible Causes: Normal heart rhythm is called sinus rhythm. The speed at which the heart beats will increase or decrease based upon the body's needs. Tachycardia, a heartbeat that is too fast, and bradycardia, a heartbeat that is unusually slow, can both be caused by issues with the nervous and endocrine systems. Bradycardia can also be a side effect of some medications. Arrhythmias can be triggered by viral illness, alcohol, tobacco, changes in posture, exercise, caffeine and recreational drug use. Sinus bradycardia is where the heartbeat is slow, but still under control, and can occur when in a state of deep relaxation.

General Signs and Symptoms: The most common symptom of tachycardia is the awareness of a fast heartbeat (palpitations). Chest pain, anxiety and shortness of breath may also be experienced. Common symptoms of bradycardia include fatigue, light-headedness and feeling faint (pre-syncope). Dizziness and fainting (syncope) can happen in both.

Conventional Medical Treatment: Treatment usually depends on the type and severity of the arrhythmia. Any underlying conditions will also need to be treated. Medication including anti-arrhythmic drugs can be prescribed. If the tachycardia is life-threatening an implantable cardioverter defibrillator (ICD) may be used to monitor the heart rate and automatically shock it into normal rhythm when required. If the bradycardia is persistent, a pacemaker may be implanted. Any medication causing bradycardia will need to be stopped.

Prognosis: The large majority of people with an arrhythmia lead a normal life, particularly if underlying conditions are well managed.

Holistic Advice: Stop smoking. Take regular exercise and eat a healthy balanced diet. Maintain a healthy weight and lose weight if necessary.

Carpal Tunnel Syndrome

Definition: Nerve compression at the wrist.

Possible Causes: Pressure on the median nerve as it passes through the carpal tunnel. The carpal tunnel is a small tunnel that runs from the bottom of the wrist to the lower palm through which several tendons pass, as well as the median nerve. The median nerve has both sensory and motor functions so it affects not only how the hand feels but how it moves. Carpal tunnel syndrome may be familial, and certain conditions such as gout, lupus, hypothyroidism, diabetes, pregnancy, obesity, rheumatoid arthritis, oedema and Lyme disease may increase its risk of developing. Keeping the hand or wrist in one position or carrying out repetitive tasks may trigger or worsen the condition. Structural abnormalities of the wrist may also cause this syndrome.

General Signs and Symptoms: Tingling, numbness or pain in the median nerve, which affects the thumb, index finger, middle finger and half of the ring finger. Pain may be worse of a night. Manually dexterity may be reduced. Moving the hand or shaking the wrist can help to alleviate the symptoms.

Conventional Medical Treatment: Symptoms may clear up without treatment. Wrist splints and corticosteroid injections can be used and, in severe cases surgery may be required to reduce the pressure on the nerve. When the condition is brought on by an underlying condition, treating that condition may help the carpal tunnel syndrome.

Prognosis: Left untreated it can lead to permanent nerve damage.

Holistic Advice: Avoid over-straining neck, arms and hands. Do not lift heavy objects. Seek regular massage to the neck and shoulders. Relax with head and neck well supported on a regular basis. Review seating position during driving and computer work. Deal with any obesity. Chiropractic may be of benefit.

Cellulitis

Definition: An infection of the deeper layers of the skin, most commonly affecting the hands, feet and lower legs.

Possible Causes: Usually caused when a bacterial infection penetrates the deeper layers of the skin. The breaks in the skin that allow the bacteria in can be caused by dryness (resulting in cracks), cuts or bites. Those who find it difficult to move around, are overweight and have poor circulation are at particular risk of developing cellulitis. Additional risk factors include previous history of cellulitis, weakened immune system, bedsores, lymphoedema and recent surgery wounds.

General Signs and Symptoms: Skin of the affected area(s) may become red, hot and painful. The skin can also swell and blister. The infection can spread to the rest of the body causing fever, high heart rate, confusion, dizziness, clammy skin and loss of consciousness. These symptoms could be indicative of sepsis, which is a medical emergency.

Conventional Medical Treatment: In mild cases, a short course of antibiotics will be prescribed. Moving the joint near the area and raising the affected body part will help reduce inflammation. Painkillers and anti-inflammatories can help to reduce pain. In recurring cases long-term antibiotics will be used to manage the condition and to stop infections coming back.

Prognosis: In mild cases, symptoms should resolve in 7 to 10 days. If not treated promptly the infection can spread to the blood, muscles and bones causing serious complications, including sepsis. Sepsis is a medical emergency and is a life threatening condition.

Holistic Advice: Take precautions, such as wearing appropriate gloves and footwear, to prevent any cuts or scrapes in the future. Keep skin clean and moisturised. Drink plenty of fluids.

Cervical Cancer

Definition: Cancer of the cervix.

Possible Causes: Human Papillomavirus (HPV) causes almost all cases of cervical cancer; most commonly strains HPV 16 and HPV 18. It is a very common virus which can be passed on through any type of sexual contact but does not always develop into cancer. Additional risk factors of developing cervical cancer include; smoking, weakened immune system, taking the oral contraceptive pill and having more than 5 children (particularly under the age of 17).

General Signs and Symptoms: In early stages, there are often no symptoms. The most common sign is abnormal vaginal bleeding occurring during/after sex and bleeding between periods. In advanced cervical cancer other symptoms such as pain in the lower back, constipation, incontinence, blood in urine, severe vaginal bleeding and swelling of the lower limbs can occur.

Conventional Medical Treatment: Dependant on the location, size and type of cancer. For early cervical cancer, surgery may be used to remove the cervix or the entire womb (hysterectomy). For advanced cancer, radiotherapy, chemotherapy and targeted therapies can be used to kill cancers cells and try to prevent them from coming back.

Prognosis: Cervical cancer is often curable if diagnosed early. Complications can occur due to the cancer and also due to the treatment received. Early menopause can be triggered if the ovaries are damaged or removed by treatment. The vagina may narrow due to radiotherapy which can make sex painful or difficult.

Holistic Advice: Using condoms during sex can offer some protection against HPV infection. Reduce risk factors by stopping smoking, seeking alternative forms of contraception and take steps to improve immune function.

Cervical Spondylitis

Definition: A form of arthritis that mainly affects the neck.

Possible Causes: Most commonly caused by age related wear and tear to the vertebrae in the neck. It is a very common condition with people over the age of 50. There is a higher risk of developing cervical spondylitis at a younger age if there has been a previous neck injury or family history of the condition. People with jobs that have repetitive neck movements or lots of overhead work are also at increased risk.

General Signs and Symptoms: Most commonly experienced are neck and shoulder pain that comes and goes. Headaches that originate from the back of the neck may also be present.

Conventional Medical Treatment: Dependent on severity of symptoms. Painkillers can be used to reduce pain. Muscle relaxants can be prescribed if the pain is chronic. Gentle exercise and stretches for the neck may be recommended. If symptoms do not improve referral to a physiotherapist could be required.

Prognosis: There is no cure but symptoms can be managed. Exercise can help maintain the range of movement and strengthen the muscles to better support the area.

Holistic Advice: Take gentle exercise and stretches for the neck.

Chilblains

Definition: Small, itchy, painful, red-purple swellings on the fingers, toes and other extremities such as the ears and nose.

Possible Causes: Excessive narrowing of blood vessels under the skin in cold weather then, as the vessels dilate when the body warms, the sudden increased blood flow causes blood to leak into the tissues. Chilblains may be acute, healing a couple of weeks after exposure to the cold, or chronic, causing persistent problems. Risk factors include poor circulation, lupus, family history, poor diet, and exposure to cold and damp environments, Raynaud's disease and smoking.

General Signs and Symptoms: Typically occur a couple of hours after exposure to the cold. The chilblains are painful when exposed to the cold and become very itchy and produce a burning sensation as the skin warms up again. The affected area may become red and swollen and in extreme cases the skin may break forming sores and blisters. Children and the elderly are most susceptible.

Conventional Medical Treatment: If the chilblains become infected antibiotics may be prescribed. Otherwise an over the counter mixture of friar's balsam and iodine can be painted on the site, lanolin ointment can be used to keep the skin supple, and antiseptic cream can help to avoid infection.

Prognosis: Chilblains do not usually cause permanent damage and will normally disappear without treatment if the affected area is protected from the cold, but they may recur. In extreme cases they may lead to infection, skin discoloration, ulcers and scarring.

Holistic Advice: Keep warm! Dress appropriately in the winter and avoid drafts. Take regular exercise to promote circulation. Stop smoking and avoid tight clothing and shoes that may restrict circulation. Do not try to reheat up the hands or feet quickly when they get cold by putting them on a heater etc. because this will speed up the sudden return of the blood and worsen the pain and the condition.

Chlamydia

Definition: A sexually transmitted infection caused by bacteria.

Possible Causes: Caused by the Chlamydia trachomatis bacteria, chlamydia is one of the most common sexually transmitted infections (STIs) in the UK. It is usually spread through unprotected sexual intercourse or contact with genital fluids. A pregnant woman can pass chlamydia to her baby.

General Signs and Symptoms: Most people with chlamydia do not realise they have it, as symptoms are often unnoticed. If symptoms do develop, most people experience pain when passing urine and unusual discharge from the penis, vagina or bottom. Women can experience pain/bleeding after sexual intercourse and men can experience pain/swelling in the testicles.

Conventional Medical Treatment: Can be effectively treated with antibiotics. Current and recent sexual partners should also be tested and treated.

Prognosis: A very high success rate with correct usage of prescribed antibiotics. If left untreated chlamydia can cause severe complications. In men, the testicles and epididymis can become inflamed (epididymitis). In women, chlamydia can spread to womb, ovaries or fallopian tubes causing pelvic inflammatory disease, which can lead to fertility issues. Chlamydia can also cause pregnancy complications such as premature birth. Both men and women can also experience reactive arthritis, but this is more common in men.

Holistic Advice: Prevention is key; use of a condom or barrier during sexual intercourse. Avoid sharing sex toys, if you do share them ensure they are covered with a condom and cleaned after use.

Chronic Obstructive Pulmonary Disorder (COPD)

Definition: An umbrella term for a group of lung conditions that cause breathing difficulties, including emphysema (damage to the air sacs) and chronic bronchitis (long term inflammation of bronchi).

Possible Causes: Smoking is the main cause of COPD. The chemicals inside the cigarette smoke can damage the sensitive lining of the airways and lungs. Smokers that have a close relative with COPD have an increased risk of developing the condition. Fumes, dust and chemicals in the workplace have also been found to damage the lungs. These include cadmium (dust and fumes), grain/flour dust, silica dust, welding fumes and coal dust. The risk of developing COPD is very high for smokers that have exposure to the above dust/chemicals/fumes.

General Signs and Symptoms: COPD is chronic and symptoms develop slowly, getting worse over time. Breathlessness (at rest and during exercise), a persistent chesty cough, frequent chest infections and wheezing are the most common symptoms. Tiredness, weight loss, swelling in the ankles and chest pain are less common but may also be present.

Conventional Medical Treatment: The aim of treatment is to control symptoms and slow progression. The most effective way of preventing COPD from getting worse is stopping smoking. Bronchodilator inhalers (short acting and long acting) are often prescribed to widen the airways and make breathing easier. If breathlessness persists, a steroid inhaler can be combined with the above. Mucolytic medicines can be used to make phlegm easier to cough up. Short courses of antibiotics are often taken if signs of a chest infection are present. An individualised exercise and education programme called pulmonary rehabilitation might be used to improve symptoms and emotional wellbeing. When symptoms are severe, a nebuliser can be used to deliver large amounts of medicine and oxygen therapy can be administered. In very few cases, surgery can be used to remove badly damaged sections of the lung.

Prognosis: There is currently no cure for COPD. Management of symptoms with a care team is key to prolonging a good quality of life. Eventually COPD will progress and become life threatening.

Holistic Advice: Stop smoking. Take prescribed medicines. Maintain a healthy body weight and take regular exercise. Try to limit exposure to environments that can cause a flare up such as cold weather, dusty places, fumes, smoke, strong smelling cleaning products and air fresheners. Practice breathing techniques.

Cirrhosis

Definition: Irreversible scarring of the liver.

Possible Causes: Healthy liver tissue is destroyed and replaced by scar tissue which starts to block the flow of blood through the liver so reducing liver function. This is usually caused by excessive alcohol consumption or the hepatitis C virus. Less common causes include hepatitis B, inherited liver disease, non-alcoholic steatohepatitis and autoimmune hepatitis. The first stage of alcoholic liver disease is known as fatty liver. Fatty liver usually reverses after 3-6 months of abstinence from alcohol. If drinking is not halted, the second stage is alcoholic hepatitis (liver inflammation). Some may still recover from this stage if alcohol is given up. Cirrhosis is the third stage and is irreversible. Women drinkers are at a greater risk of developing cirrhosis, although cirrhosis affects more men than women (because more men drink heavily). Please refer to drinkaware.co.uk for the current safe drinking guidelines for men and women.

General Signs and Symptoms: The early stages of cirrhosis often pass symptom-free. However, after several years of heavy drinking the scar tissue builds up and the liver begins to lose function. The resulting symptoms include loss of appetite, weight loss, discomfort in the upper-right side of the abdomen, tiredness, nausea and very itchy skin. In later stages of cirrhosis there are many symptoms including jaundice, oedema, vomiting blood, tendency to bruise easily, rapid heartbeat, breathlessness, dark, tarry faeces and a build up of fluid in the legs and abdomen. Ultimately the liver may fail.

Conventional Medical Treatment: Cirrhosis cannot be cured so the treatment focuses on preventing it from progressing and managing the symptoms. The treatment depends on the cause. If due to alcohol, lifestyle changes must be made. If due to an underlying disease such as viral hepatitis or autoimmune hepatitis, medication can be given. The treatment given to ease the symptoms will depend on the symptoms being experienced. The only treatment for liver failure is a liver transplant.

Prognosis: The outlook depends on the severity of the liver damage. Many can live with cirrhosis for many years, but it can lead to liver cancer and liver failure.

Holistic Advice: Cirrhosis can be largely avoided by drinking within the guidelines, and taking precautions to avoid infection from the hepatitis B and C viruses.

Coeliac Disease

Definition: An autoimmune condition where the immune system attacks its own tissues causing damage to the small intestine.

Possible Causes: The exact cause of coeliac disease is unknown. When gluten is ingested, the immune system produces an abnormal reaction releasing antibodies, which mistakenly attack healthy cells and tissues of the small intestine. Damage to the healthy cells decrease the absorption of nutrients in the small intestine. Gluten is found in food such as cereals, bread and pasta. Factors known to increase the risk of developing coeliac disease are family history, digestive system infections in childhood and having a very early introduction to gluten as a baby (before 3 months). Having other health conditions such as type 1 diabetes, thyroid conditions, ulcerative colitis, epilepsy, Down's syndrome and Turner syndrome may also increase the risk of coeliac disease however it is unknown if the conditions are directly responsible.

General Signs and Symptoms: Symptoms tend to come and go and it is unknown why some people suffer mildly and some people suffer severely. The most common symptom is diarrhoea caused by poor absorption of nutrients in the small intestine. In addition, abdominal pain, bloating, indigestion, constipation and flatulence may be experienced. Fatigue, balance issues, tingling and numbness in the hands and feet as well as weight loss and fertility issues are also potential symptoms of coeliac disease. Those with coeliac disease often develop an itchy rash called dermatitis herpetiformis.

Conventional Medical Treatment: Those with coeliac disease will need to adopt a gluten-free diet. Referral to a dietician to help create a personalised, balanced diet is an important step to managing this condition. Sometimes supplements of vitamins and minerals may be encouraged whilst the digestive system is going through repair.

Prognosis: A well-maintained gluten-free diet should relieve symptoms within a couple of weeks. It could take up to two years for the digestive system to fully heal depending on the amount of damage sustained. If not treated, coeliac disease can result in malabsorption and malnutrition. Malabsorption can cause anaemia, vitamin B12 and folate deficiency and osteoporosis. Malnutrition can cause severe fatigue, muscle wastage and confusion.

Holistic Advice: Eat gluten free food and follow a balanced gluten free diet. Check the labels of food to ensure they are gluten-free. Unsafe food items include bread, pasta, cereals, biscuits, cakes, pies, gravies and sauces unless they are labelled as gluten-free.

<u>Cold Sore</u>

Definition: An inflamed blister usually found in or around the mouth.

Possible Causes: Viral infection by the Herpes simplex virus, specifically Type 1 HSV. Initial exposure usually occurs infants or young children after skin to skin contact with someone who has a cold sore. After initial infection, the virus lays dormant in the skin and can be triggered to reoccur by minor trauma to the area, the common cold, sun exposure, menstruation and stress. Often there may be no trigger for recurrence.

General Signs and Symptoms: Initial signs include tingling, itching or burning in the area where the eruption is about to occur. Within the next 48 hours a small fluid filled blister will usually appear. These are most commonly found around the mouth but can appear anywhere on the face. As it heals, the blister may burst and scab becoming itchy and painful. Cold sores are very contagious during the initial tingling period prior to eruption and during the healing period.

Conventional Medical Treatment: Mild eruptions often require no treatment. Blisters can be covered using a cold sore patch. Antiviral creams can be used for more severe infections and to speed the healing process. Topical creams can be used to soothe irritation and painkillers can be taken for pain.

Prognosis: A lifelong condition. The large majority of cases resolve within 10 days. The virus can be spread to other parts of the body causing eye or throat infections as well as further skin conditions such as eczema herpeticum. People with compromised immune systems are at particular risk of further complications.

Holistic Advice: Drink plenty of fluid. Do not touch the cold sore. Wear high factor lip balms when in the sun. Wash your hands regularly particularly before and after applying any creams. Try to avoid triggers for your cold sores. Try to boost the immune system.

Colitis

Definition: Inflammation of the inner lining of the colon (large intestine).

Possible Causes: Many potential causes including bacterial or viral infection (e.g. campylobacter, E.coli and salmonella), loss of blood supply to the colon, inflammatory bowel diseases (Crohn's and Ulcerative Colitis), allergic reaction and microscopic colitis.

General Signs and Symptoms: Symptoms can depend on the cause and may include abdominal pain, bloating and cramping. Diarrhoea is a key indicator of colitis and blood may or may not be present. Additional symptoms include fever, chills, fatigue and dehydration. If caused by Crohn's disease or ulcerative colitis there may be other symptoms such as joint swelling, mouth ulcers and skin inflammation.

Conventional Medical Treatment: Treatment dependant on the cause. Rehydration is important and can be achieved through drinking fluids or intravenously in severe cases of dehydration. Changes to the diet can be beneficial to reduce flare-ups. If the cause is an inflammatory bowel disease then various medications may be used to reduce inflammation.

Prognosis: Some bacterial infections that cause colitis can resolve without any treatment. If caused by inflammatory bowel diseases then lifelong management of symptoms will be required.

Holistic Advice: Keep a diary to see if any foods worsen the condition. Drink plenty of fluids.

Colorectal Cancer

Definition: Cancer that is found in the large intestine or rectum. Also known as bowel cancer.

Possible Causes: Exact cause is unknown but there are risk factors that increase the chance of developing the disease including being over the age of 60 and having a family history of bowel cancer. Other chronic bowel conditions such as ulcerative colitis and Crohn's disease are also linked to bowel cancer. Lifestyle factors including being overweight or obese, a diet high in processed meat and low in fibre, smoking, alcohol consumption and being inactive all increase the risk of developing bowel cancer.

General Signs and Symptoms: The three most common symptoms include persistent changes to normal bowel habits (increased need to poo, constipation or looser poo), persistent blood in the poo and persistent lower abdominal pain that is always caused by eating. Unintentional weight loss, tiredness, and a lump in the abdomen or rectum may also be experienced.

Conventional Medical Treatment: Dependent on the size, type and location of the cancer. Surgery can be used for cancer located in the large intestine and in the rectum. A stoma may be required to allow the remaining bowel to heal after surgery. This may be a temporary or permanent measure depending on the circumstances. Chemotherapy and radiotherapy can both be used to destroy cancer cells and to help prevent them from returning. Targeted cancer medication can also be used to slow the growth of the cancer

Prognosis: Dependent on the size, type and location of the cancer. Treatment for bowel cancer can permanently change the way the bowel functions causing changes to bowel habits, looser poo or having difficulty emptying the bowel fully.

Holistic Advice: Lose weight if required and eat a healthy balanced diet. Stop smoking and reduce alcohol consumption. Take regular exercise.

Common Cold

Definition: A viral infection of the upper respiratory tract. Also referred to as a cold.

Possible Causes: Most commonly caused by a large group of viruses called rhinoviruses. Easily spread directly through close contact with people via expelled droplets in the air. Droplets can also land on objects and spread the virus indirectly when a person touches the object and proceeds to touch their eyes, nose or mouth.

General Signs and Symptoms: Symptoms often appear gradually, mainly affect the nose and throat and can linger for 1 – 3 weeks. A blocked/runny nose (non-allergic rhinitis), sneezing, sore throat and a cough are typical symptoms. In some cases muscle aches, fever and loss of taste and smell are experienced.

Conventional Medical Treatment: The large majority of cases will not need any medical intervention and can be treated at home. A blocked nose can be relieved with decongestant sprays or medicines. Paracetamol or ibuprofen can be used to reduce any fever or pain.

Prognosis: Full recovery within a few weeks.

Holistic Advice: Drink plenty of fluids, keep warm and rest. To reduce the chances of getting or transmitting a cold, practice good hand hygiene, exercise regularly and eat a heathy balanced diet.

Concussion

Definition: Temporary injury to the brain. Also known as a mild traumatic brain injury.

Possible Causes: Acute trauma in the form of a bump, blow or jolt to the head.

General Signs and Symptoms: Usually occur within minutes or hours of head injury. Less commonly, symptoms take a few days to show. Signs of concussion include a headache that cannot be relieved with painkillers, dizziness, nausea, vomiting, memory loss, loss of balance, feeling stunned/dazed/confused, vision disturbances and struggling to stay awake. If, after head injury, there are problems with memory, persistent headache, repeating vomiting, changes in behaviour **and** the person has been drinking alcohol or has taken recreational drugs they should attend their nearest A&E department.

Conventional Medical Treatment: Dependent on severity of injury and symptoms. Mild concussion can usually be treated at home with rest. Paracetamol/ibuprofen for headache and avoidance of alcohol can both aid recovery. More severe injury to the head should be assessed in hospital to rule out serious brain injury.

Prognosis: Dependent on the severity of the injury. Most people feel better within a few days or weeks. On some occasions, symptoms can last months. This is known as post-concussion syndrome and includes ongoing headaches, dizziness, memory issues, problems with balance, depression and anxiety. Repeated concussions have been linked to serious brain conditions such as chronic traumatic encephalopathy.

Holistic Advice: Take precautions to reduce the chance of head injury such as wearing a seatbelt when driving, wearing a helmet when riding a motorbike, bicycle or horse. When participating in sport ensure the use of recommended safety equipment. Avoid contact sport or strenuous exercise for at least 3 weeks post injury. Only gradually increase activity when symptoms have reduced.

Congenital Heart Disease

Definition: One or more defects of the heart that are present from birth. There are two main types – cyanotic and acyanotic. When the heart defect results in too little oxygen in the blood, it is called cyanotic heart disease. In acyanotic heart disease, there is sufficient oxygen in the blood but the defect in the heart prevents the blood from being circulated correctly.

Possible Causes: Congenital heart disease is the most common birth defect but the cause of the abnormal foetal development is largely unknown. It can sometimes run in families, indicating a genetic link. Congenital heart disease may also be associated with genetic disorders such as Down's syndrome. Exposure of the foetus to excessive alcohol and drugs may increase the risk. If the mother contracts certain infections (e.g. rubella) in early pregnancy, or is diabetic, there is an increased likelihood that the baby will be born with this condition. Septal defects (commonly called hole in the heart), in which there is a hole in the wall that divides the left and right sides of the heart, is one of the most common defects. Atrial septal defects occur between the two 'collecting' chambers of the heart and allow extra blood to flow into the right side of the heart, causing it to enlarge. Ventricular septal defects occur between the two 'pumping' chambers of the heart and allow extra blood to flow to the lungs, increasing lung pressure. Heart valves, the aorta and other blood vessels may be defected, and in some cases there may be multiple defects.

General Signs and Symptoms: Many defects result in a shortness of breath, breathing difficulties, difficulty in feeding, poor appetite, sweating, chest pains, slow weight gain and delayed growth. If the defect causes low oxygen levels in the blood, the tongue and lips may appear blue and it may cause fainting.

Conventional Medical Treatment: There is a variety of surgical techniques to correct the defect. About half of babies born with congenital heart disease will require immediate surgery. The remainder will probably require surgery or medication at some later point in childhood.

Prognosis: Depends on the type of heart defect and its severity. Even very severe defects can often be successfully corrected. 85% of children born with a heart defect will live to reach adulthood.

Holistic Advice: It may be possible to reduce the risk a little by the mother taking good care of herself during pregnancy.

Constipation

Definition: The infrequent, difficult or incomplete emptying of the bowel which leads to hard faeces.

Possible Causes: Can be caused by a number (and often a combination) of factors including insufficient fibre and fluids in the diet, changes in routine and eating habits, lack of exercise and immobility, anxiety and depression, and ignoring the urge to defaecate. Drinking too much alcohol and caffeine is dehydrating which makes the faeces harder and more difficult to pass. Can also be caused by some medications (e.g. antacids, antidepressants and diuretics) and is common in pregnancy. It can be symptomatic of an underlying medical condition such as colon or rectal cancer, diabetes, hypothyroidism, some nervous system disorders and irritable bowel syndrome.

General Signs and Symptoms: Less frequent or more difficult defaecation of dry, hard and lumpy faeces. Constipation can also cause stomach aches and cramps, bloating, nausea and loss of appetite.

Conventional Medical Treatment: Lifestyle changes in diet, exercise and routine may enable the condition to be relieved without the use of medication. Laxatives can be given to promote defaecation. For more serious cases suppositories and enemas may be required. Treatment is usually effective but it may take several months to re-establish regular bowel movements. Any underlying condition needs to be identified and treated appropriately.

Prognosis: Many will only experience constipation for a short time, with no impact on health. Cases of chronic constipation can cause significant pain and discomfort. It can lead to hard faeces remaining in the rectum, and liquid faeces leaking around it causing diarrhoea.

Holistic Advice: Drink plenty of water and eat a healthy, low fat but high fibre diet. Try to adopt a routine of opening the bowel at the same time every day and try not to resist the urge to defecate. Take regular exercise and reduce stress to help the functioning of the digestive system.

<u>Contact Dermatitis / Eczema</u>

Definition: A condition that causes inflammation of the skin (derma- = skin, -itis = inflammation). Eczema is also known as dermatitis, although we often (incorrectly) only tend to associate eczema with atopic dermatitis, which is the most common and hereditary form of eczema and mainly affects children. Atopic dermatitis is linked to other conditions such as asthma and hay fever. We'll concentrate on contact dermatitis here. Remember it is still a type of eczema.

Possible Causes: Can be caused by allergies or irritants. Allergic contact dermatitis is caused by exposure to a substance that causes an abnormal reaction from the immune system (e.g. cosmetics, some plants, metals such as nickel or cobalt in jewellery). Irritant contact dermatitis is caused by contact to a substance that damages the skin (e.g. chemicals, detergents, perfumes, dust). Irritants are the most common cause. Stress and poor diet may play a part.

General Signs and Symptoms: Inflammation, itching, redness, dryness, cracking, blistering, scaling and weeping of the skin, crusts and secondary skin infections. Most common on the hands and face.

Conventional Medical Treatment: The best treatment is to try to avoid the allergen or irritant. Emollients, creams, lotions and ointments can be used to soften and soothe skin. In more severe cases corticosteroids may be prescribed for topical application. Any secondary infection can be treated with antibiotics. If the dermatitis fails to respond to the treatments mentioned above, a dermatologist can prescribe alitretinoin tablets. They can be prescribed only by a dermatologist because they can cause serious side effects and must be carefully monitored.

Prognosis: Dermatitis can usually be successfully managed but in some cases can have a severe and long lasting affect on quality of both personal and working life.

Holistic Advice: Ensure a good balanced diet of fresh fruit and vegetables. Drinking plenty of water can help to keep the skin hydrated. Hypoallergenic moisturisers may be of benefit. Try to avoid exposure to potential allergens and irritants. If exposure occurs, wash the affected skin as soon as possible. If exposed to irritants at work ensure employer is informed of condition and any personal protective clothing provided is used.

Corns and Calluses

Definition: Areas of hard, thickened skin on the hands or feet.

Possible Causes: Prolonged pressure or friction on a small area of skin. Badly fitting shoes is a major contributing factor to the development of corns and those with misshapen feet are particularly susceptible. Calluses can be caused by repetitive actions that produce pressure on the feet such as jogging, or an uneven distribution of body weight. Musicians may get calluses on their fingers due to friction from guitar strings etc.

General Signs and Symptoms: There are 2 main types of corn. Hard corns are the most common. They show as small circles of hard skin with a clear centre, usually on bony parts of the toes. Soft corns are whitish and rubbery in texture and are usually found in areas between the toes. They can be extremely painful and are subject to infection due to their moist location. Calluses are yellowy, rough, usually painless areas of hard skin, occurring on areas of the feet and hands subjected to excess friction.

Conventional Medical Treatment: Removing the source of pressure or friction is a priority. Corn pads can be used to keep the pressure off a hard corn and a variety of toe separators and special plasters is available. A Doctor or Chiropodist may be able to cut off some of the hard callused skin or reduce the size of the corn by paring it down. Calluses can be gradually removed by soaking the feet in warm water and then gently rubbing them with a pumice stone.

Prognosis: Once the callus or corn has been removed it should not return providing that the source of the pressure or friction is also eliminated. Corns and calluses may become infected and ulcerated, particularly in those with diabetes. If this occurs, medical help should be sought.

Holistic Advice: Wear shoes that fit. Wash the feet regularly and dry them properly. Moisturising the feet with special foot cream may help. Change socks or tights every day.

Cor Pulmonale

Definition: Impairment to the right ventricle of the heart as a result of respiratory disease. The right ventricle becomes enlarged and pumps blood less effectively until it fails. Also known as right-sided heart failure.

Possible Causes: The most common causes are pulmonary hypertension and chronic obstructive pulmonary disease (COPD). Cor pulmonale can also be acute (sudden) and caused by venous thromboembolism which is an obstruction of a blood vessel by a blood clot that has become dislodged from another area in the body's circulatory system. Other lung diseases such as emphysema, pneumoconiosis and cystic fibrosis can cause this condition. Neuromuscular disorders that cause chronic hypoventilation like polio, myasthenia gravis and motor neurone disease can also cause cor pulmonale.

General Signs and Symptoms: Early symptoms are often non specific and can include breathlessness or rapid breathing, fatigue, worsening cough and chest pain. Swelling of the feet and ankles, coughing up blood, blue colouration of the skin and a hyper expanded chest may also present.

Conventional Medical Treatment: Rapid treatment of the underlying lung condition. Oxygen therapy may be required. Diuretics may be required to reduce the presence of oedema (swelling). If caused by thromboembolism, anticoagulation medication may be prescribed. In severe cases, a heart or lung transplant might be recommended.

Prognosis: Dependent on the underlying cause and its rate of progression.

Holistic Advice: Stop smoking. Maintain a healthy weight and eat a balanced diet. Take regular exercise.

Coronary Thrombosis

Definition: Formation of a blood clot within a blood vessel(s) of the heart.

Possible Causes: Thrombus in the blood vessels of the heart is most commonly caused by atherosclerosis (see page 31). This is where fatty deposits clog the arteries, causing the vessels to harden and narrow.

General Signs and Symptoms: Symptoms do not usually arise until the blood flow becomes restricted or blocked. In the case of coronary thrombosis, blood flow restriction will lead to a heart attack. Heart attack is characterised by sudden onset of severe, crushing pain in the centre of the chest. This may spread up to the neck and into the arms. The skin becomes pale and there is sweating and shortness of breath. Overwhelming anxiety is often experienced. Heart attacks can occur without chest pain.

Conventional Medical Treatment: Can be treated with medicine or surgery. Coronary artery bypass graft (CABG) to divert blood around the blocked artery can be performed. Alternatively, a stent can be inserted to widen the artery (angioplasty). Statins (for high cholesterol), medicine to lower the blood pressure and reduce the risk of blood clots may also be prescribed.

Prognosis: Risks can be managed and reduced with medicine and lifestyle changes. Heart attack is a potentially life-threatening condition.

Holistic Advice: Eat a healthy balanced diet and take regular exercise. Maintain a healthy weight and lose weight if necessary. Stop smoking and reduce alcohol consumption.

Cough

Definition: A reflex response to an infection or irritation of the respiratory tract.

Possible Causes: Acute coughs are commonly caused by a viral infection of the respiratory tract, such as the common cold, flu, laryngitis or bronchitis. Allergic conditions (e.g. hay fever) may also cause a cough. The respiratory tract can also be irritated by mucus and inhaled irritants such as dust and smoke which cause the reflex action. Coughs can also be caused when small objects, typically pieces of food, are accidentally inhaled. Chronic coughs can be caused by smoking, underlying conditions (e.g. asthma, rhinitis and gastro-oesophageal reflux) and can be a side effect of some medicines (e.g. ACE inhibitors). Occasionally a cough can be a symptom of a more serious condition (e.g. lung cancer and heart failure).

General Signs and Symptoms: There are 2 main types of cough. A dry cough feels like a constant tickle in the throat and no phlegm is produced. A chesty or productive cough (usually as a result of infection) feels deeper and phlegm may be produced. The chest and ribs may become sore with the exertion of coughing and, because sleep may be affected (coughs tend to be worse when lying flat), the sufferer may feel tired and achy.

Conventional Medical Treatment: Cough medicines may help to relieve the symptoms. For dry coughs, cough suppressants may be used. For chesty coughs, expectorants may help bring up the phlegm so that coughing becomes easier. Antibiotics serve no purpose for viral infections, but may be prescribed if there is a secondary bacterial infection. If the condition persists, investigations such as X-rays or lung function tests may be required to ensure there is no serious underlying condition.

Prognosis: Most coughs only last a few days to a couple of weeks. If the cough produces bloody mucus or causes chest pain or shortness of breath, medical advice should be sought.

Holistic Advice: Lemon and honey drinks are useful to soothe the throat. Steam inhalation may help to loosen the mucus. Anything that can boost the immune system will be of benefit because the cough (if viral) will remain until the body defeats it.

Cramp

Definition: Sudden painful contraction of a muscle.

Possible Causes: Most cramps have no underlying cause, but they can be brought on by vigorous exercise, which causes an accumulation of lactic acid in the muscle. Excessive sweating can also lead to a loss of sodium which often causes cramp. Cramp may also be associated with poor circulation, or triggered by swimming in cold water, over-tiredness and tension. Occasionally, cramp may be an indication of an underlying disease such as motor neuron problems, metabolic problems such as liver, kidney or thyroid conditions, and dehydration. Certain medications may also induce leg cramps, e.g. diuretics, statins (used to lower blood-cholesterol levels) and some asthma drugs.

General Signs and Symptoms: Painful and sudden contraction of muscle, commonly in the legs. The calf is most often affected but the thigh and feet can get cramp too. Cramp can cause a lack of mobility and normally lasts only for a few seconds. After and episode of cramp, the muscle will often feel hard and painful and remain sore for several hours.

Conventional Medical Treatment: Because there is usually no underlying cause, treatment is very limited. Due to the speed and duration of the attacks, painkillers are unlikely to be of benefit. In some cases, quinine has shown to have benefits but more research is necessary, particularly regarding any side effects. Self-help is likely to be the best route. Stretching the muscles and massaging the affected muscle can bring relief.

Prognosis: Although unpleasant and sometimes very painful, cramp is not likely to cause any lasting damage. Exercises to stretch the muscles can help to prevent cramp as well as ease it out when it strikes.

Holistic Advice: For night cramp, keeping the feet warm can help, so use bed socks or place the feet on a feather pillow (which holds body heat and does not go cold like a hot water bottle). Supporting the toes while asleep may also help. A regular massage can be of benefit because it may stimulate the circulation and lymphatic system, helping to release tension and waste products from the muscles.

Crohn's Disease

Definition: A chronic inflammatory disease that can affect any part of the digestive tract.

Possible Causes: The exact cause is unknown. There may be a genetic factor, because there is more chance of developing Crohn's disease if close relatives have it. It may be caused by a malfunction in the immune system, causing the body to attack "friendly bacteria" in the intestines, and various environmental factors are also thought to play a part. Smokers are twice more likely to develop this disease than non-smokers, and their symptoms are often more severe.

General Signs and Symptoms: Areas of the digestive tract become inflamed. Any part of the digestive tract can be affected but it is most commonly found in the ileum and the colon. Inflammation often occurs in more than one part of the tract, with unaffected or mildly affected areas between. The inflammation can cause diarrhoea, abdominal pain, fever, weight loss and a general feeling of ill health. If the colon is affected the stools may contain blood and there may be some rectal bleeding. Episodes may be severe, lasting weeks or even months, before settling down to show only mild (or no) symptoms. Usually begins in early adulthood and can cause serious ill health throughout life.

Conventional Medical Treatment: Mild attacks can be treated with antidiarrhoeal drugs. For an acute attack steroids are commonly prescribed. Severe cases may need hospitalisation. Aminosalicylate drugs (to reduce persistent inflammation of the intestines) and immunosuppressant drugs may be prescribed to help reduce the frequency of the attacks. Dietary supplements may be required to counter any malabsorption. Most sufferers will need surgery at some stage to remove the diseased area.

Prognosis: Symptoms tend to recur despite treatment and the condition is lifelong. Complications such as intestinal obstruction, ulcers, fistulae (passageways that develop and run from the bowel), and malabsorption problems may occur. There is also a significantly increased risk of developing colorectal cancer.

Holistic Advice: Keep a food diary to see if any foods worsen the condition.

Cushing's Syndrome

Definition: Hormonal disorder associated with high levels of steroid hormones.

Possible Causes: Constantly high levels of steroid hormones in the blood. This could be due to long term treatment with steroid medication for another illness (e.g. asthma or arthritis), or a disorder that causes the overproduction of cortisol (e.g. pituitary or adrenal tumours).

General Signs and Symptoms: Sudden weight gain, bloating around the chest and stomach, red and rounded face, excessive growth of facial or body hair (especially in women), irregular menstruation or amenorrhoea, reddish-purple stretch marks on the abdomen, thighs, buttocks, breasts, arms and legs, oedema, heavy sweating, muscle wasting and weakness, tendency to bruise easily, wounds slow to heal, acne, loss of libido, depression and mood swings. Some may experience headaches, high blood pressure, high blood glucose level, an increased thirst and an increased need to urinate.

Conventional Medical Treatment: If it is caused by taking steroid medication for another illness, it may be possible to reduce the dose and seek alternative treatments. If the body is producing too much cortisol, cortisol-inhibiting drugs may be used. If the symptoms are caused by a tumour, the tumour may be removed by surgery, radiotherapy or chemotherapy, all of which have possible serious complications.

Prognosis: May be cured but recovery is slow. Untreated it can lead to complications such as high blood pressure, thinning of the bones, diabetes mellitus and chronic heart failure.

Holistic Advice: Never alter the dose of any prescribed drug without first consulting a doctor.

Cuts and Abrasions

Definition: A cut, or laceration, is an area of skin that has been fully broken with a sharp edge. An abrasion, or graze, is where the top layers of skin have been scraped off.

Possible Causes: Cuts can occur anywhere on the body and are most commonly caused by trauma with a penetrative object such as a sharp knife or piece of glass. Abrasions commonly occur due to a fall and the knees, elbows and hands are often affected.

General Signs and Symptoms: The skin is fully broken or torn in the instance of a cut. The wound will often bleed and may gape in the middle. Cuts can be clean with straight edges or jagged with uneven edges depending on how the trauma occurred. Abrasions are superficial and can be painful but bleeding is often minimal. In both cuts and abrasions, during the healing process, a scab may form over the wound to allow new skin to grow underneath. Cuts and abrasions can easily become infected bringing symptoms of swelling or redness around the wound and fever. Pus may be present and the glands of the neck, armpits and groin may swell.

Conventional Medical Treatment: Most minor wounds can be treated at home. Initial treatment should focus on stopping any bleeding from the cut or abrasion. With minor or small wounds, pressure can be applied with a clean absorbent material. It is beneficial to raise the affected area above the heart if possible. Once the bleeding is stopped the wound should be cleaned with water, pat dried with a clean towel and covered with a sterile adhesive dressing such as a plaster. Dressings can be changed as often as necessary. Painkillers can be taken for pain or inflammation. Medical attention should be sought if the bleeding cannot be stopped, there is a loss of skin sensation around the wound, there is something stuck in the wound or if there are signs of infection. Infection will be treated with antibiotics.

Prognosis: Minor cuts and abrasions begin to heal within a few days. There is risk of infection if the cut or abrasion has been contaminated with dirt or there is something stuck under the skin.

Holistic Advice: Keep the wound clean and covered during the initial healing process. Do not pick at any scabs that form.

Cystic Fibrosis

Definition: An inherited condition that causes mucus to build up in the lungs and digestive system.

Possible Causes: Cystic fibrosis is inherited genetically and is present from birth. A faulty gene affects the movement of water and salt both in and out of the cells. Alongside recurrent infections, this causes a build-up of thick sticky mucus in the lungs and digestive system. Both parents must have a copy of the faulty gene in order to pass the condition onto their child. The parents may not have cystic fibrosis themselves and only carry a copy of the gene that causes it.

General Signs and Symptoms: The build-up of mucus in the lungs can cause breathing difficulties and increase the risk of lung infections. Reoccurring chest infections, wheezing, coughing, shortness of breath and abnormally widened airways (bronchiectasis) are all common symptoms. Mucus can also build up in the pancreas, causing issues with digestion that can lead to malnutrition. Jaundice, diarrhoea, constipation and difficulty putting on weight are common. Bowel obstruction can occur in newborn babies.

Conventional Medical Treatment: Treatments aim to control symptoms, prevent complications and improve quality of life. Medicines to reduce or thin the mucus produced and bronchodilators to widen the airways can be prescribed. Antibiotics will be used to treat any chest infections. A physiotherapist can teach airway clearance techniques such as ACBT (active cycle of breathing techniques), autogenic drainage and the use of airway clearance devices. Regular exercise is encouraged. In severe cases, as a last resort, a lung transplant may be recommended. Dietary advice will be given to ensure enough calories are being consumed as well as the correct amounts of vitamins and minerals. Digestive enzyme capsules may be recommended to aid digestion.

Prognosis: There is currently no cure for cystic fibrosis but symptoms can be managed with treatment. Over time the condition will worsen, causing a reduced life expectancy. There is a susceptibility to infection and a high chance of developing complications. People with cystic fibrosis are more likely to develop other conditions such as osteoporosis, diabetes, nasal polyps, liver problems and fertility problems.

Holistic Advice: Eat a healthy, balanced diet as advised by the health care team. Exercise regularly.

Cystitis

Definition: Inflammation of the bladder. Because the bladder is a part of the urinary tract, cystitis is classed as a urinary tract infection (UTI).

Possible Causes: Usually it is a result of a bacterial infection which causes inflammation of the bladder lining. Bacterial infection can be caused by not emptying the bladder fully (so harbouring bacteria), and by bacteria entering the urethra from the anal or vaginal areas and then traveling up to the bladder. Cystitis can also be caused by the irritation or damage to the area around the urethra. The can be caused by factors such as frequent or vigorous sex, wearing tight clothing and chemical irritants. It can also be symptomatic of some underlying conditions such as other bladders problems, kidney conditions and, in males, prostatitis. People with diabetes mellitus are more likely to suffer from urinary tract infections because the presence of glucose in the urine may encourage bacterial growth.

General Signs and Symptoms: The most common symptoms are an urgent and frequent need to urinate, and pain or stinging when passing urine. Other symptoms include dark, cloudy or strong smelling urine, a feeling of incomplete emptying of the bladder, blood in the urine, and lower abdominal pain. The sufferer may feel generally unwell, weak and feverish. Cystitis is more common in women than men and more frequent if the woman is pregnant, sexual active or post-menopausal.

Conventional Medical Treatment: Mild cystitis can often be cleared up by drinking plenty of water and taking painkillers such as paracetamol and ibuprofen. More serious infections may need antibiotics.

Prognosis: Most cases clear up on their own, but some do not respond to antibiotics and the sufferer may experience many recurring episodes. It is also possible for the infection to move to the kidneys. In a few severe cases, there can be a complete or partial loss of bladder control as a result of the irritation of the muscle in the bladder wall.

Holistic Advice: Avoid synthetic underwear, tights and close fitting trousers. Drink plenty of water and cranberry juice. Do not use any perfumed products around the genitals. Empty the bladder frequently and completely, after going to the toilet wipe from front to back, wash before and after sex, and urinate after sex. Avoid coffee, food containing vinegar, citrus fruits and spicy foods as these may trigger the condition.

Dandruff

Definition: Common condition that affects the scalp causing flakes of skin to appear.

Possible Causes: It is associated with the accelerated renewal of skin cells, which causes more dead skin to be shed. Sensitivity to yeasts that are produced naturally by the body can cause dandruff, and not brushing hair regularly results in the dead skin cells not being physically removed. Excessive dandruff is known as seborrhoeic dermatitis, which causes the skin to become inflamed and flaky, and results in larger, greasier flakes.

General Signs and Symptoms: White flakes of skin on the scalp and in the hair. Head may feel sore, greasy or itchy. Affects men more than women, often after puberty.

Conventional Medical Treatment: Dandruff shampoos and scalp preparations can be used to control the condition. Antifungal shampoos inhibit the growth of the fungi and yeasts. In severe cases the GP may prescribe steroid scalp applications to reduce the inflammation.

Prognosis: Responds well to treatment but can reoccur at any time.

Holistic Advice: Although not caused by poor hygiene, it can affect self-esteem. Ensure hair is rinsed properly after washing and brush hair regularly. Avoid using chemicals on the scalp. Try to keep well hydrated to avoid the skin from drying.

Deep Vein Thrombosis

Definition: Formation of a blood clot within a deep lying vein, usually in the leg. Often abbreviated to DVT. Also called venous thrombosis.

Possible Causes: Usually caused by a combination of slow blood flow through a vein, an increased tendency of the blood to clot, and a damaged vein wall. Risk factors include long periods of immobility (e.g. during a long air flight or if confined to bed), pregnancy, accidental injury to a blood vessel, surgery, family history of thrombosis, being overweight, smoking, dehydration and taking the combined oral contraceptive pill.

General Signs and Symptoms: Pain or tenderness in the leg, swelling of the lower leg or thigh, enlarged veins below the skin, heavy ache in the affected limb and redness and heat in the affected area.

Conventional Medical Treatment: Anticoagulants, such as heparin and warfarin, may be used to help prevent the clot getting bigger and to reduce the risk of further clots developing. Compression stockings can help prevent the calf from swelling and reduce the pain. Only rarely is surgery used to remove a clot. Raising the leg above the hip helps to relieve the pressure on the vein.

Prognosis: DVT is not usually dangerous in itself, but there is a risk that a fragment of the clot could break off and lodge in a pulmonary artery, causing a pulmonary embolism. A history of DVT may lead to post-thrombotic syndrome, causing long term symptoms such as calf pain, swelling, a rash in the affected area and (in severe cases) ulcers.

Holistic Advice: Try to avoid long periods of inactivity. Stretch and move regularly. Take regular exercise, lose any excess weight, don't smoke and eat a healthy diet. Drink plenty of water.

Dementia

Definition: A syndrome and a group of related syndromes associated with an ongoing decline of brain function. Includes Alzheimer's disease, vascular dementia, dementia with Lewy bodies and frontotemporal dementia.

Possible Causes: Many of the diseases associated with dementia are caused by an abnormal build up of proteins in the brain. This build up causes nerve cells to function inefficiently and ultimately die. Alzheimer's disease is the most common type of dementia and is thought to be caused by a build up of the proteins amyloid and tau. The second most common cause of dementia is vascular dementia. This is caused by restricted blood flow to the brain by narrowing/blockage of blood vessels, a single stroke or lots of 'mini' strokes. Mixed dementia is where Alzheimer's and vascular dementia occur at the same time. Lewy bodies are small protein clumps that damage the way brain cells communicate, causing them to die. It is closely related to Parkinson's disease. Frontotemporal dementia is more common in younger people and is caused by clumping of proteins in the front and temporal lobes. It is more likely to run in families than other causes of dementia. Much rarer causes of dementia or dementia like symptoms are Huntington's disease, corticobasal degeneration, progressive suprenuclear palsy and normal pressure hydrocephalus.

General Signs and Symptoms: Symptoms vary depending the area of the brain that is damaged. People will experience symptoms in their own way. Common early symptoms that appear before dementia diagnosis include memory loss, difficulty concentrating, becoming confused with daily tasks, time and places, struggling with conversation and mood changes. Memory issues are most common with Alzheimer's disease. Vascular dementia can have stroke-like symptoms (muscle weakness and temporary paralysis) and movement problems as well as memory issues. Lewy bodies cause many of the symptoms of Alzheimer's as well as hallucinations, slow physical movements, repeated falls and fluctuating levels of alertness/drowsiness. Frontotemporal dementia can cause personality changes, lack of social awareness, language problems and obsessive behaviours such as over eating and drinking. The most common symptoms of the later stages of dementia include difficulty remembering loved ones, communication issues (including losing the ability to speak), mobility issues, behavioural issues (including aggression and wandering), bladder incontinence and difficulty eating/drinking.

Conventional Medical Treatment: The majority of the medicines available are to treat Alzheimer's due to it being the most common form of dementia. Various drugs can be prescribed to slow the loss of mental function. Other conditions such as stroke, heart problems, diabetes and hypertension affect the symptoms of vascular dementia. These conditions should be diagnosed and treated. Depression and sleeping problems may be relieved by antidepressants. Cognitive stimulation therapy (CST) involves group activities to help improve memory and language ability in mild to moderate dementia.

Prognosis: There is no cure, but treatment can slow the progression of the disease.

Holistic Advice: Brain function can be helped by not smoking or drinking large quantities of alcohol, taking regular exercise, eating a balanced, healthy diet, and keeping the brain stimulated by learning new skills and participating in activities.

Depression

Definition: Feelings of sadness, often accompanied by loss of interest in life and reduced energy. It is one of the most common mental health disorders. Specific types of depression exist, including seasonal affective disorder, postnatal depression, and bipolar depression (formally known as manic depression), in which there are periods of depression and periods of excessively high mood (mania).

Possible Causes: There is no single cause. It can be triggered by a stressful event (or more commonly a combination of stressful events) such as bereavement, divorce, illness, and job and money worries. Risk factors include certain conditions such as coronary heart disease, cancer, and head injuries, low self esteem, family history of depression, traumatic event in childhood, giving birth, social isolation, drinking alcohol and taking drugs. Women are more likely than men to become depressed but, given that the suicide rate in men is higher, this could be because men are less likely to seek help for their depression.

General Signs and Symptoms: Feeling of sadness or misery that lasts most of the day. Common symptoms include loss of interest and motivation, low energy, tearfulness, poor concentration, low self-esteem, feeling worried or anxious, feelings of guilt, difficulty in making decisions, insomnia, unexplained aches and pains, loss of hope, changes in appetite and weight, and decreased sex drive. There may be thoughts about self-harm or suicide. Depression can interfere with working, social and family lives.

Conventional Medical Treatment: Mild depression can often spontaneously lift. Antidepressants may be prescribed and psychosocial treatments (such as counselling and cognitive behavioural therapy) used. For severe depression, electroconvulsive therapy or lithium may be recommended. Depression may recur if antidepressant drugs are withdrawn too soon.

Prognosis: With the right treatment and support, most make a full recovery.

Holistic Advice: Take regular exercise and maintain a balanced, health diet. Try to talk about feelings with others. Relaxation techniques and breathing exercises may help, as may engaging in a distracting hobby. Support groups can offer advice and information, as well as providing a forum to openly discuss feelings with those who have had similar experiences. There are many self-help resources to help with depression. Always remember that depression is a serious illness, not a weakness.

Diabetes Insipidus

Definition: Disorder caused by the body's inability to control its water balance. Not related to diabetes mellitus, although both conditions cause thirst and the excessive passing of urine.

Possible Causes: The amount of water in the body is regulated by antidiuretic hormone (ADH). In this condition either too little is produced (cranial diabetes insipidus) or the body fails to respond to its effect (nephrogenic diabetes insipidus). This results in too much urine being passed which, in turn, causes the extreme thirst. The most common cause of cranial diabetes insipidus is damage to the hypothalamus caused by a brain tumour, brain surgery or a head injury. It may also be caused by the immune system attacking brain tissue. Other causes include cancers that spread to the brain, brain infections that cause damage and conditions that suddenly reduce the blood supply to the brain (e.g. stroke). Nephrogenic diabetes insipidus may be congenital or acquired. The most common cause of acquired nephrogenic diabetes insipidus is taking certain medications (e.g. lithium (used for bipolar disorder)). Other causes include having too much calcium in the blood or too little potassium, and kidney damage caused by infection or obstruction.

General Signs and Symptoms: There is a persistent thirst and the frequent need to pass a large quantity of pale, dilute urine. These symptoms can affect sleeping patterns, causing tiredness and irritability. Sufferers may feel generally unwell.

Conventional Medical Treatment: Treatment aims to reduce the quantity of urine passed. Cranial diabetes insipidus may be treated with a drug called desmopressin that mimics antidiuretic hormone. Thiazide diuretics may be used to increase the concentration of the urine which, in these cases, decreases the output. Non-steroidal anti-inflammatory drugs may also help. Nephrogenic diabetes insipidus may be treated by a change of medication. A change of diet is also commonly required. Thiazide diuretics and non-steroidal anti-inflammatory drugs may be prescribed in severe cases. It is important to drink sufficiently so as not to become dehydrated.

Prognosis: Outlook depends on the cause.

Holistic Advice: Sufferers should carry identification to alert others of the condition in case of emergency.

Diabetes Mellitus

Definition: Diabetes is a chronic condition caused by too much glucose in the blood. There are 2 main forms - diabetes insipidus (caused by the hyposecretion of antidiuretic hormone) and diabetes mellitus (caused by the hyposecretion of insulin). There are 2 types of diabetes mellitus - type 1 and type 2 (see below).

Possible Causes: The amount of sugar in the blood is controlled by insulin. Insulin helps to move glucose from the blood into the cells to be broken down to release energy. Type 1 diabetes occurs when no insulin is produced. Type 1 usually occurs suddenly in childhood and is often referred to as juvenile diabetes or early-onset diabetes. It is thought to be an autoimmune condition in which the cells of the pancreas are attacked. This may be triggered by a viral infection, and there may be a familial link. In type 2 diabetes, either too little insulin is secreted or the body's cells become resistant to it, and so the glucose in the blood in not fully utilized. About 95% of all diabetics have this type. It develops slowly but the exact cause is not known. The risk of type 2 diabetes increases with age and is linked to obesity. Ethnic origin may be a factor (African-Caribbean or south Asian origins are more at risk) and it appears to be familial.

General Signs and Symptoms: Deposits of sugar in the urine, extreme thirst and a dry mouth, increased urination, constipation, lack of energy, dehydrated skin, recurring thrush, blurred vision, cramps, muscle weakness, loss of weight, skin infections and poor circulation, which can result in wounds being slow to heal. If the blood sugar becomes very low, a "hypo" attack may occur causing the sufferer to feel shaky, sweaty, weak, sick and confused.

Conventional Medical Treatment: The aim of treatment is to keep blood glucose levels as normal as possible. Type 1 diabetes is treated with insulin injections and so is often referred to as insulin dependent diabetes. Type 2 can usually be controlled at first by adapting the diet and making lifestyle changes. If the blood glucose level creeps up, oral medicines can be given to reduce it but insulin injections may be required ultimately. A hypo attack is treated by giving sugar orally or a glucagon injection to raise the blood glucose level.

Prognosis: There is no cure and it is a lifelong condition. Complications can cause eye, kidney, cardiovascular and nervous system problems. Blood glucose levels, blood pressure and cholesterol levels should be regularly monitored.

Holistic Advice: Exercise regularly and lose excess weight. Don't smoke. Only drink alcohol in moderation. A usual healthy diet that is high in fibre, fruit and vegetable and low in fat, salt and sugar is advised. Diabetes dietitians offer specific advice. Take care of the feet and eyes, and information cards should be carried or a bracelet worn if prone to unstable blood sugar levels.

Diarrhoea

Definition: The passing of frequent, loose watery stools.

Possible Causes: Diarrhoea is not a disease in itself but may be a symptom of an underlying condition. Short (acute) bouts, especially if accompanied by vomiting, are often caused by gastroenteritis. Gastroenteritis is commonly caused by a viral infection (e.g. norovirus) or bacterial infection (e.g. E.coli and salmonella). Those with reduced immunity are more susceptible to infectious gastroenteritis. Other causes of acute diarrhoea include emotional upset, taking antibiotics, and drinking too much alcohol or coffee. Chronic diarrhoea, lasting more than 2 weeks, can also be due to a viral or bacterial infection, but can also be caused by the use of laxatives, poor diet, or can be symptomatic of an underlying intestinal disorder, e.g. ulcerative colitis, irritable bowel syndrome, Crohn's disease and lactose intolerance.

General Signs and Symptoms: Diarrhoea may be accompanied by abdominal pain, bloating, loss of appetite and vomiting. Can lead to dehydration, causing headache, weakness and lethargy.

Conventional Medical Treatment: Usually clears up within a couple of days. Drink plenty of water. Associated symptoms tend to clear when rehydrated. Rehydration drinks can help rebalance the salt and sugar levels. Antidiarrhoeal drugs can help reduce the bowel movement but are not always advised. Painkillers can help any fever or headache. If caused by an underlying intestinal disorder, the disorder will be addressed.

Prognosis: Usually temporary, but if prolonged the underlying cause must be established. Dehydration can be dangerous, particularly in babies, children and the elderly.

Holistic Advice: The risk of developing infectious gastroenteritis (and therefore diarrhoea) can be reduced by washing the hands regularly, particularly after going to the toilet and before eating.

Diverticular Disease

Definition: The presence of small pouches known as diverticula in the wall of the colon that cause the symptoms associated with this disease.

Possible Causes: Pea-sized pouches form when parts of the intestine (usually the lower colon) bulge outwards. The bulging is often associated with persistent constipation. It is estimated that by the age of 50, 50% of people will have diverticula. If the diverticula are causing no symptoms, it is called diverticulosis. When the presence of these pouches causes symptoms, it is called diverticular disease. When the pouches become infected and inflamed (possibly by a hard piece of faeces getting trapped in the pouch, allowing bacteria to develop) the condition is called diverticulitis. Risk factors may include low-fibre diet, smoking, obesity, having a history of constipation, physical inactivity, and the use of non-steroidal anti-inflammatory drugs (e.g. ibuprofen).

General Signs and Symptoms: Diverticular disease can cause episodes of abdominal pain (especially in the lower left abdomen) and bloating that is relieved by defaecation or the passing of wind. There may be intermittent bouts of constipation and diarrhoea, and occasional bright red bleeding from the rectum. Diverticulitis can cause a more persistent, severe lower abdominal pain, tenderness in the abdomen, fever, nausea, vomiting, painful or frequent urination, and rectal bleeding.

Conventional Medical Treatment: Often a high-fibre diet with plenty of fluids is the only treatment required for diverticular disease. Paracetamol tends to be recommended for the abdominal pain. Diverticulitis may require antibiotics to treat any bacterial infection. Surgery may be required to remove the diseased part of the colon if severe bouts of diverticulitis occur frequently.

Prognosis: Diverticular disease can usually be controlled and does not have serious associated complications. However, with diverticulitis, the inflamed diverticula can burst, allowing faeces and blood to spill into the abdominal cavity. This can lead to peritonitis (the inflammation of the lining of the abdomen), which can be fatal if not treated quickly. There is also the risk of abscesses, fistulae (passageways that develop and run from the bowel) and intestinal obstruction.

Holistic Advice: Drink plenty of fluids and eat a high-fibre diet. Any changes in bowel movement or rectal bleeding should be reported to a Doctor as it can indicate a serious underlying disease.

Drug Misuse

Definition: The use of a substance that is not consistent with legal or medical guidelines. Drugs can be legal or illegal and used recreationally, dependently or for medical reasons.

Possible Causes: There are many reasons why people chose to use drugs. Misuse becomes a problem when a person uses drugs in a way that is harmful to their health and wellbeing.

General Signs and Symptoms: Dependent on the drug, the amount taken, how the drug is taken and how often the drug is taken. Sedative drugs such as alcohol, heroin and tranquilisers depress the nervous system and can give feelings of warmth, relaxation and provide short term relief of physical and/or emotional pain. Withdrawal from regular use or dependency can cause flu like symptoms including aches, sweating, chills and spasms. Stimulants such as amphetamine, cocaine and ecstasy give a rush of energy, increasing heart rate and body temperature. Chronic overuse of stimulants can cause insomnia, restlessness, weight loss, anxiety, paranoia and hyperactivity. Prescription drugs are used for medical purposes but are also open to misuse. Prescription drug dependency can manifest itself as mood swings or irritability based on drug availability, disturbed sleeping patterns, frequent doctors' visits and defensiveness around medications. Work or school performance may be implicated and there may be increasing disinterest in personal appearance.

Conventional Medical Treatment: Dependent on the drug, if the person wants to control or abstain from drug taking and if dependency is present. Treatment can be given at home or at a rehabilitation facility. Talking therapies such as cognitive behavioural therapy can be used to identify any emotional reasons behind the misuse. Self-help groups are often advocated. Medicines can be used as a substitute for dependency on opioid drugs whilst other treatments are on-going. Detoxification or detox is for people who want to stop their drug taking completely and will assist with withdrawal.

Prognosis: Abstinence will have the greatest health benefits. It is very important to set realistic targets under any treatment plan. Long-term drug misuse can have serious complications such as organ damage, psychoses and even death. Sharing needles when injecting drugs increases the risk of vein damage, abscesses and infection including HIV and hepatitis.

Holistic Advice: Set realistic targets under any treatment plan.

Dysmenorrhoea

Definition: Pain associated with menstruation.

Possible Causes: In most cases the pain is a normal part of the menstrual cycle, caused by muscular contractions of the uterine wall. This is called primary dysmenorrhoea and there may be a familial link. In some cases, dysmenorrhoea is caused by an underlying medical condition such as endometriosis, fibroids, pelvic inflammatory disease, adenomyosis (when the uterine lining grows into the muscular layer of the uterus) and having an intrauterine contraceptive device fitted. This is called secondary dysmenorrhoea.

General Signs and Symptoms: Pain and/or painful cramping in the lower abdomen. The pain may radiate to the lower back and legs. Other symptoms may include headache, nausea, tiredness, dizziness and diarrhoea. The symptoms usually begin just before or at the start of menstruation, with the pain being worst when the bleeding is heaviest.

Conventional Medical Treatment: Primary dysmenorrhoea may be treated with over-the-counter non-steroidal anti-inflammatory drugs (e.g. ibuprofen and aspirin) or other pain killers such as paracetamol. The use of the combined contraceptive pill may also help to reduce symptoms. In cases of secondary dysmenorrhoea, the underlying condition will be treated. Once under control, the dysmenorrhoea usually disappears.

Prognosis: Can usually be successfully treated.

Holistic Advice: Taking hot baths or applying a source of heat to the abdomen (e.g. hot water bottle) may provide relief. Gentle exercise may help to reduce the pain. Light circular massage around the abdomen may be helpful. Relaxation techniques may also be of benefit.

Dysuria (Painful Urination)

Definition: A symptom of pain, discomfort or burning when urinating.

Possible Causes: The most common cause of painful urination are urinary tract infections (UTI) which can occur in the kidney, ureter, bladder and urethra. Sexually transmitted infections (STI) such as genital herpes, chlamydia and gonorrhoea can also cause painful urination. Both UTIs and STIs are caused by bacteria entering the urinary tract. General inflammation and irritation to the urinary tract from sexual activity, passing stones, interstitial cystitis, vaginal changes due to menopause, scented hygiene products and side effects from certain medications can also cause dysuria. Risk factors increasing the chance of developing painful urination include being female, diabetes, advanced age, enlarged prostate, kidney stones, pregnancy and having a urinary catheter.

General Signs and Symptoms: Pain, discomfort or burning when urinating. Additional symptoms that can accompany dysuria include fever, increased urge to urinate, abnormal discharge, abdominal pain and lower back pain. Changes may also occur to the normal flow of urine as well as the colour, amount and clarity due to the presence of blood or pus.

Conventional Medical Treatment: Determine the underlying cause.

Prognosis: Once the underlying cause has been determined and treated, the dysuria should stop completely.

Holistic Advice: Drink plenty of water. Seek medical advice if your urine changes in appearance or causes you pain/discomfort.

Ear Problems

General Information: Disorders of the ear are very common and in severe cases may interfere with communication, causing significant disability. As well as being the organs of hearing, the inner ear also contains structures that help to maintain balance and so disorders of the ear can lead to symptoms such as dizziness. Below is a brief summary of 5 common ear conditions.

Deafness: Partial or total loss of hearing in one or both ears. May be congenital, or caused by disease, injury or age. Deafness that results from the failure of the outer ear to transmit sound to the inner ear is often temporary, e.g. when the middle ear fills with fluid following infection or wax, or sudden changes in air pressure. Damage to the part of the inner ear that detects sound or to the nerve tends to cause permanent deafness, e.g. noise-induced hearing loss or Ménière's disease (a disorder of the inner ear causing sudden episodes of severe dizziness, nausea and hearing loss). Hearing aids are commonly used to help correct permanent deafness.

Earache: Pain originating in the ear. It can be caused by a wide range of ear disorders, infections and blockages, but can also be caused by the build up of mucus after a cold or toothache.

Glue Ear: Childhood condition in which fluid builds up in the middle ear. It causes temporary, partial deafness but usually gets better without medical intervention.

Tinnitus: Sounds, often ringing, buzzing or whistling, that originate from one or both ears. The sounds may vary in volume, and episodes can be brief but in some it is permanent. Cause is often unknown but can be associated with ear disorders such as Ménière's disease and noise-induced hearing loss. It may also be a symptom of an underlying medical condition, e.g. anaemia and hyperthyroidism. Masking devices can be used that produce sounds to distract from the tinnitus. It can be very distressing, leading to depression and anxiety.

Vertigo: A false sensation of movement, often combined with nausea and vomiting. It may be impossible to walk or even stand. Vertigo often develops suddenly, lasting a few seconds to several days. It is caused by a disturbance in the inner ear resulting from many factors including arthritis in the neck (that affects blood flow to parts of the brain associated with balance), inner ear infections, Ménière's disease, excess alcohol, heatstroke and food poisoning. Lying still will help in the short term. The underlying cause must be identified for persistent episodes.

Ectopic Pregnancy

Definition: When a fertilised egg implants itself outside of the womb.

Possible Causes: Incorrect implantation of a fertilised egg, usually in the fallopian tubes. In many cases, the exact cause is unclear. Risk of ectopic pregnancy is increased by pelvic inflammatory disease, previous ectopic pregnancy, previous surgery on the fallopian tubes, infertility treatment (such as IVF), becoming pregnant whilst using implanted contraception, smoking and age.

General Signs and Symptoms: Symptoms usually develop between the 4th and 12th week of pregnancy and can include a combination of the following; a missed period and/or positive pregnancy test, one-sided lower abdominal, watery discharge and vaginal bleeding, discomfort when going to the toilet and pain in the tip of the shoulder (could indicate internal bleeding). In severe cases, the fallopian tube may rupture causing a medical emergency. Symptoms of a rupture include sudden, sharp, intense abdominal pain, dizziness, nausea and pale skin.

Conventional Medical Treatment: There are three treatments available for ectopic pregnancies. Expectant management is used when the ectopic pregnancy is expected to resolve naturally, the symptoms are mild (low levels of pain and light bleeding) and the pregnancy is very small. This consists of regular blood tests to monitor hormones. If expectant management is not suitable medication may be given via injection to stop the pregnancy from developing. In many cases, keyhole surgery under general anaesthetic is required to remove the pregnancy before it becomes too large. This may require the removal of the affected fallopian tube. In the case of a rupture, surgery is required to repair the fallopian tube as quickly as possible.

Prognosis: Unfortunately, it is never possible to save the pregnancy. Reliable contraception will be required for at least 3 months after the use of medications to stop the pregnancy from developing, as the drug is harmful for the baby if pregnancy occurs. If surgery is required, recovery can take around 4 – 6 weeks however, it is believed that fertility is not adversely affected.

Holistic Advice: Stop smoking. If a pregnancy is possible and you have a combination of any of the above symptoms seek medical advice as quickly as possible.

Emphysema

Definition: Progressive damage to the lungs, resulting in wheezing and shortness of breath. Sufferers also usually have chronic bronchitis and the resulting condition is called chronic obstructive pulmonary disease (COPD).

Possible Causes: In emphysema the alveoli in the lungs become enlarged and damaged, making them less efficient in transferring oxygen to the blood stream. In chronic bronchitis the bronchi become inflamed, congested and narrowed, obstructing the flow of air. Smoking is the most common cause. Air pollution, passive smoking, and occupational exposure to fumes, dust and other lung irritants, can be contributory factors. Smokers with a sibling with COPD are at a higher risk of developing the disease, and there is a rare genetic condition that causes a deficiency of a protein that protects the lungs, so increasing the risk of COPD.

General Signs and Symptoms: Difficulty breathing, wheezing and shortness of breath. The symptoms build up gradually, getting worse over time. There tends to be a persistent productive cough, an increase in sputum production and frequent chest infections. Cold weather and infections such as flu worsen the condition. Some sufferers of emphysema may develop a barrel-shaped chest as the lungs distend. It is more common in men although the incidence in women is rising.

Conventional Medical Treatment: Damage to the lungs caused by COPD is irreversible. Preventing further exposure by making lifestyle changes as soon as possible is the only way to limit further damage. Treatment can only help ease the symptoms. Bronchodilator drugs can help make breathing easier, mucolytic drugs can help thin the mucus to make it easier to cough up. Antibiotics may be used to help treat chest infections and steroids may be prescribed for a bad flare-up. In severe cases nebulisers (to administer medicine in vapour form through a face mask) and oxygen therapy may be required. If fluid builds up in the tissues, diuretics may be prescribed.

Prognosis: It can result in respiratory failure, reduced kidney function and heart failure. Fewer than 1 in 20 people with COPD live longer than 10 years after diagnosis.

Holistic Advice: Stop smoking. Take gentle exercise. Vaccinations against flu and pneumonia may be recommended.

Endometriosis

Definition: The presence of endometrium cells (the cells that line the interior wall of the uterus) in other parts of the body, such as the fallopian tubes, ovaries, bladder, bowel, vagina and rectum.

Possible Causes: The endometriosis cells outside of the womb go through a menstrual pattern in the same way as the endometrium. However, when these cells break down causing a bleed, the blood is trapped in the body. This can lead to pain, swelling and tissue damage. The cause is not known for definite, but it may be caused by fragments of the endometrium which, when shed during menstruation, do not leave the body as normal, but instead travel along the fallopian tubes, possibly enter the pelvic cavity and attach to organs. It may also be the case that endometriosis cells travel to other parts of the body by accessing the blood or lymphatic systems. It may also be caused by a combination of genetic, immune system, hormonal and environmental factors.

General Signs and Symptoms: Pain in the lower abdomen, pelvis or lower back, particularly before and during menstrual periods. Menorrhagia (excessive menstrual flow), dysmenorrhoea (painful menstruation) and irregular menstruation are common. Sufferers may have a lack of energy, depression, fertility problems and experience pain during sexual intercourse. The pain varies according to where the cells are located.

Conventional Medical Treatment: In mild cases the condition may get better by itself. The pain can be reduced with non-steroidal anti-inflammatories and pain killers. Hormone treatments can be given for several months to limit or stop the production of oestrogen and so prevent menstruation. This may help reduce the endometriosis. Surgery can be used to remove or destroy areas of endometriosis tissue, depending on where the tissue is located. In severe cases, a hysterectomy and the removal of the ovaries plus any areas of endometriosis may be suggested.

Prognosis: It is a chronic condition with no cure but symptoms can usually be managed successfully. Infertility is the greatest problem and, although some treatments may increase fertility, getting pregnant can often be problematic. Adhesions on the ovaries may also lead to ovarian cysts. Endometriosis may recur until the menstrual cycle ends at the menopause, but is unlikely to recur if the ovaries are removed.

Holistic Advice: Relaxation exercises can be useful to help to cope with the pain.

Epilepsy

Definition: A disorder of brain function causing recurrent seizures.

Possible Causes: Seizures are symptomatic of abnormal electrical activity in the brain. There are 3 main types. 1. Symptomatic - when there is a known cause (e.g. brain injury, drug or alcohol abuse, meningitis, stoke and brain tumour). 2. Idiopathic – when there is no known cause. 3. Cryptogenic – when there is no known cause but there is evidence (such as learning disorders) to suggest that it may be due to brain damage. Triggers may include stress, lack of sleep, fever, low blood-sugar level, and flashing lights.

General Signs and Symptoms: Seizures vary from a few seconds in a trance-like state, to convulsions and total loss of consciousness. Seizures are categorized according to how much of the brain is affected. In a partial seizure, only a part of the brain is affected but a generalised seizure affects all (or most) of the brain. Partial seizures may be simple or complex. In a simple partial seizure, consciousness is maintained but the head and eyes may turn to one side, the muscles in the arms, legs and face may stiffen, and one side of the body may twitch. There may be tingling sensations, muscle weakness and strange sensory sensations. In a complex partial seizure, the person may enter an uncommunicative state. They may smack the lips, grimace and fidget, and have no memory of the seizure. A generalised seizure may render the person unconscious and often leads to a fall. There are several types including absences (loss of awareness, most common in children), myoclonic jerks (muscle twitches), clonic seizure (longer lasting twitching), atonic seizure (causing all the muscles to relax), tonic seizure (causing all the muscles to stiffen) and tonic-clonic seizure. Tonic-clonic seizure is the most common form of epilepsy. It is typified by body stiffness, twitchy limbs, loss of consciousness and urinary incontinence. Epileptics may be able to feel the onset of an episode

Conventional Medical Treatment: Most cases can be successfully treated with anti-epileptic drugs. Failing that, vagus nerve stimulation may be considered. A device is implanted that stimulates the vagus nerve in the neck. This has been shown to reduce the frequency and severity of the attacks. Brain surgery is only used if the part of the brain affected is small and its removal would not cause a significant loss of brain function.

Prognosis: There in no cure but treatments can usually control the condition.

Holistic Advice: Because stress may trigger an attack, exercise and relaxation exercises such as yoga and meditation may help. Avoid all triggers.

Eye Problems

General Information: Many eye disorders do not affect sight but a few serious conditions may damage the structures of the eye and lead to loss of vision. Eye disorders are common and early diagnosis tends to lead to successful treatment.

Cataract: Clouding of the lens of the eye, causing blurred or distorted vision. The cataracts are caused by structural changes to protein fibres in the lens, resulting in the cloudy appearance. They can be congenital but are most common after the age of 75. They usually develop in both eyes but one can be more severely affected. Risk factors for cataracts in the young are eye injury, prolonged exposure to sunlight, diabetes mellitus, or long term use of corticosteroids. The cataract can be surgically removed and an artificial lens put into the eye.

Corneal Ulcer: A deep erosion of the cornea. Corneal ulcers can be very painful and, if left untreated, can cause scarring and lead to permanently impaired vision, blindness or even loss of the eye. They can be caused by injury and/or infection. Symptoms include intense pain in the eye, redness and discharge from the eye, and an increased sensitivity to light. People who wear contact lenses are at increased risk. Antibiotics or antiviral drugs may be prescribed to treat the infection, which usually clears up with 1-2 weeks.

Glaucoma: Abnormally high pressure of fluid inside the eye. This is caused by a blockage of the fluid as it tries naturally to flow out of the eye. The rise in pressure may cause damage to the nerve fibres in the retina (the light-sensitive part of the eye) and the optic nerve causing permanent damage. It mainly affects those over 60 and is familial. Glaucoma can be acute (developing suddenly, causing severe pain and rapid loss of vision) or chronic (developing painlessly over several years). It is diagnosed by measuring the eye pressure. Eye drops can be used to reduce the pressure. In some cases surgery may be needed to help the fluid drain. Successful treatment normally minimizes further vision loss but if left untreated it can cause blindness.

Female Infertility

Definition: Inability of a woman to conceive with a partner of normal fertility.

Possible Causes: There are 3 main stages to conception – ovulation, egg transport and fertilization, and implantation. Infertility can be caused by problems with any of these, but is most commonly caused by problems with ovulation. Conditions such as polycystic ovary syndrome, premature menopause, thyroid disorders, and some chronic conditions (such as cancer) may affect ovulation. Damage to the fallopian tubes and uterus affect successful egg transport, fertilization and implantation. Damage can be caused by a variety factors, including pelvic or cervical surgery, fibroids, endometriosis, and pelvic inflammatory disease. Risk factors include stress, excessive exercise, low body weight, obesity, some medications, age, sexually transmitted infections, smoking, and exposure to some chemicals.

General Signs and Symptoms: Inability to conceive despite having regular unprotected sex.

Conventional Medical Treatment: Medication can be given to encourage ovulation, surgical procedures may be used to help correct any anatomical problem, and assisted conception techniques, such as intrauterine insemination and in-vitro fertilization, can help sperm to fertilize the egg. When fertility can not be helped by any of the above treatments, it may be possible to receive donated eggs.

Prognosis: Treatments significantly increase the chance of pregnancy, but the success rates vary depending on the cause of infertility and the treatment given.

Holistic Advice: Infertility can put much stress on the woman and the relationship, which can then have the knock on effect of further reducing the chances of conception. Try to reduce stress, use relaxation techniques, take regular, gentle exercise, eat a balanced diet, maintain a healthy weight, stop smoking, and avoid alcohol and illegal drugs. Folic acid supplements may be advised.

Fibroids

Definition: Non-cancerous tumours that grow slowly within the muscular wall of the uterus or around the uterus.

Possible Causes: Fibroids are abnormal growths of muscular and fibrous tissue, occurring singly or in groups. Fibroids can vary in size from the size of a pea to the size of a melon. They are found in about 1 in 4 women of child bearing age and are more common in African-Caribbean people. The cause of fibroids is unknown, but they are thought to be linked to the response of the uterus to oestrogen. This link is likely to be the reason why fibroids tend to grow at times of high oestrogen level and shrink after the menopause when the oestrogen level falls. The likelihood of fibroids increases with obesity.

General Signs and Symptoms: Many with small fibroids do not display any symptoms. The symptoms of larger fibroids may vary according to their size and location. Fibroids may cause prolonged and heavy menstrual bleeding, abdominal pain, abdominal swelling, back pain, the need to pass urine frequently, constipation, and pain or discomfort during sex.

Conventional Medical Treatment: Small fibroids may not need treatment but should be checked regularly to monitor any growth. Medication can be given to reduce oestrogen levels and to treat heavy menstrual flow. A hysterectomy may be necessary in cases of large fibroids and heavy bleeding. Fibroids may also be removed by a procedure called myomectomy, the lining of the uterus can be removed by endometrial ablation, and the blood vessels that feed the fibroids can be blocked in a procedure called uterine artery embolisation.

Prognosis: Generally fibroids shrink and disappear on their own, but sometimes they can cause pain and heavy bleeding and therefore require treatment. They can affect fertility.

Holistic Advice: Eat a balanced low-oestrogen diet and exercise regularly. Acupuncture and the Bowen Technique may be of benefit.

Fibromyalgia

Definition: A chronic (long term) condition that causes pain all over the body. Also called fibromyalgia syndrome.

Possible Causes: Exact cause is unknown but it has been shown that suffers of fibromyalgia have a problem with the way in which pain messages are carried, have lower than normal levels of the hormones serotonin, noradrenaline and dopamine, and experience sleep problems. Triggers may also include physical or psychological trauma, viral infections, depression, metabolic disturbances such as an under-active thyroid, and inflammatory diseases such as rheumatoid arthritis. There may also be a genetic predisposition to this condition.

General Signs and Symptoms: Although the literal definition of the condition indicates pain (-algia) just in fibrous tissues (fibro-) and muscles (my-), the usual continuous pain extends all over the body, coupled with extreme fatigue. The condition may cause hyper-sensitivity to pain, so that even the slightest touch is painful. Stiffness, muscle spasms, poor quality of sleep, cognitive problems, headaches, and irritable bowel syndrome can also be associated. Severity of the symptoms may be affected by factors such as changes in the weather, stress levels and physical activity. Understandably, this condition often leads to depression. Affects women more than men, usually between the ages of 30-60 years

Conventional Medical Treatment: Currently no cure. Antidepressants, painkillers, muscle relaxants, anticonvulsants, antipsychotics, and medication to promote sleep can help alleviate the symptoms. Counselling-based therapies and lifestyle changes to promote good sleeping habits and relaxation can help, as may a tailored exercise programme.

Prognosis: For most the condition is permanent, but the symptoms vary in severity.

Holistic Advice: Network groups for this condition may be of use. Acupuncture, physiotherapy and treatments to aid relaxation may be of benefit. Balance periods of activity with periods of rest, don't overdo it, and rest when need to.

Flatulence

Definition: Passing of gas from the digestive system out of the anus.

Possible Causes: Every time food, drink or saliva is swallowed a small amount of air is ingested too. Gas is also released during the digestive process. This gas builds up in the digestive system and is released either through the mouth by belching or through the anus by flatulence. Food stuffs containing unabsorbable carbohydrates create more gas than other food. This is because these carbohydrates are not absorbed by the small intestine during the digestive process but get passed down to the colon where they get broken down by bacteria. This process produces gas. Foods that are high in unabsorbable carbohydrates include beans, cabbage and cauliflower. Some medical conditions can cause flatulence, e.g. constipation, irritable bowel syndrome, coeliac disease and lactose intolerance.

General Signs and Symptoms: Flatulence is a normal biological process and is only usually considered to be troublesome if there are frequent bouts of excessive wind and if the wind is considered to have a particularly unpleasant odour.

Conventional Medical Treatment: A dietary change is usually sufficient. Charcoal tablets can be purchased over-the-counter. The charcoal absorbs gas from the digestive system and so reduces flatulence.

Prognosis: Not considered to be harmful but if excessive flatulence occurs with other symptoms such as abdominal pain, bloating, episodes of constipation or diarrhoea, incontinence or blood in the stools, medical advice should be sought as it may be indicative of an underlying medical condition.

Holistic Advice: Smoking and chewing gum increases the amount of air swallowed, so avoiding these may help. Take regular exercise to promote a healthy digestive system. Peppermint tea may help.

__Folliculitis__

Definition: Inflammation of one or more hair follicles.

Possible Causes: Bacterial infection is the most common cause, but this is often preceded by physical damage to the follicle (e.g. friction, insect bite, shaving, blocked follicle). Sometimes associated with anaemia.

General Signs and Symptoms: Itchy or painful redness. Small red pimples develop in the upper part of the follicles which may then crust over. It can develop in any hairy areas of the body but is more common on the scalp, legs, buttocks, groin and armpits. In severe cases the infection may move further down into the skin creating larger areas of inflammation, even causing boils and widespread cellulitis (the bacterial infection of the dermis and subcutaneous layers of the skin). When present on the beard area of the face, folliculitis is known as Barber's itch. Pseudofolliculitis barbae is a disorder that occurs if curly beard hairs are cut too short, causing the hairs to curve back into the skin causing damage and subsequent inflammation.

Conventional Medical Treatment: Antiseptic lotions, creams and soaps are often sufficient to treat mild cases. Antibiotic creams applied topically can help to fight the infection. Antibiotic tablets may be required for stubborn infections.

Prognosis: Responds well to treatment. In severe cases it can cause scarring and, if the follicle is damaged, permanent hair loss.

Holistic Advice: Try to avoid further damage and irritation to the susceptible areas. Take extra care to ensure the infection is not spread by thoroughly cleaning equipment (e.g. razors) that makes contact with the vulnerable areas.

Foot Disorders

General Information: Feet are a weight bearing part of the body. Disorders affecting the feet can affect mobility and posture, and so have a knock-on affect to other parts of the musculoskeletal system. Here is a summary of 5 common skeletal foot disorders:

Bone Spur: A bone spur is an excessive formation of bone on normal bone. It is usually caused by localised inflammation, which triggers bone cells to deposit in the area. Spurs may cause pain if they rub surrounding tissue, and are commonly found in the back of the heel or the sole of the heel.

Club Foot: Congenital deformity of the ankle and foot. The foot (or both feet) points down and inwards. In mild cases no treatment will be necessary, but otherwise a technique called the Ponseti Method may be used to manipulate the foot into a better position and it is then set in a cast until the next manipulation is required. Surgery may also be needed to release the Achilles tendon.

Flat Feet: No space or only a little space between the foot and the ground under the medial longitudinal arch when standing. Also referred to as fallen arches. This can cause the foot to roll over to the inner side. It can be congenital but can also be caused by arthritis, a ruptured tendon, and muscular and nervous disorders. It can cause foot pain and stiffness but can often be corrected by wearing specially fitted insoles. Surgery may be required.

Foot Drop: The inability to raise the front part of the foot due to muscle weakness or paralysis caused by an underlying problem. When walking, the sufferer either drags the toes or has to lift the knee higher than normal to avoid doing so. It can be temporary or permanent, depending on the cause.

Hammer Toe: Deformity of the toe in which the end is bent downwards, so looking claw-like. Can be congenital or appear over time, sometimes caused by ill-fitting shoes. Initially it may be helped by exercising the joint to try to maintain and restore movement, but once it stiffens surgery may be necessary if it causes a problem.

High Arch: The opposite of flat foot, but much less common. The medial longitudinal arch is higher than usual, often causing pain. It is usually caused by a skeletal or nervous disorder.

Fractures

Definition: A break or crack in a bone. A simple (or closed) fracture is a clean break that has not damaged any surrounding tissues. A compound (or open) fracture is when the surrounding tissue and skin is damaged creating an open wound. A greenstick fracture is when the bone bends and breaks on the outside and not all the way through. They most commonly occur infancy/childhood due to softer bones. An impacted fracture is where the broken bones are forcefully driven into each other. A complicated fracture is where the surrounding tissues (organs, blood vessels, nerves) are significantly damaged.

Possible Causes: Fractures are commonly caused by a bone being subjected to abnormal force due to, for example, a fall or accident. The bones weaken with age and so in later life bones break easier. Diseases such as osteoporosis cause bones to thin and therefore make them more prone to fractures. Bone strength can also be decreased by certain infections, tumours and cysts. Fractures caused by underlying disease are called pathological fractures. Repeated small stresses and strains can cause stress fractures, common in athletes.

General Signs and Symptoms: Pain, swelling, misshapen body part, inability to bear weight, a grinding sound or sensation, or bleeding (in the case of an open fracture or complicated fracture). The pain and shock may cause the sufferer to look pale, clammy and feel dizzy or sick.

Conventional Medical Treatment: The bones need to be realigned and held in place for the healing process to be effective. The bone may be able to be manipulated into shape or surgery may be required to reset the bone. Bones are commonly held in place by plaster casts, but other means such as plates, rods, pins etc, can be used externally and internally as appropriate.

Prognosis: Most bones that have been successfully realigned and immobilized for up to about 8 weeks heal successfully. Physiotherapy may be required afterwards to help rebuild muscular strength.

Holistic Advice: Bone strength can be helped by ensuring a balanced diet that includes calcium. Good sources of calcium include milk, cheese, yoghurt and green leafy vegetables. Vitamin D, formed naturally by the skin when exposed to sunlight, helps the body to absorb calcium. Vitamin D is also found in eggs and oily fish. Weight-bearing exercise can help strengthen the bones. Give up smoking.

Frozen Shoulder

Definition: Pain and restriction of movement in the shoulder joint.

Possible Causes: The capsule of the shoulder joint thickens, swells and tightens, making movement difficult and painful. The cause is not always known, but it can be due to inflammation resulting from an injury, or long-term immobility. It is more common in women than men and most frequently affects those between the ages of 40-60. Risk factors include diabetes, heart disease, lung disease, hyperthyroidism, Parkinson's disease and stroke.

General Signs and Symptoms: Pain and stiffness in the shoulder joint. The condition usually starts with aching and stiffness and then it causes severe pain. The stiffness worsens and muscle tone can be lost due to the lack of movement. The pain may radiate to the elbow and be worse of a night.

Conventional Medical Treatment: Painkillers or non-steroidal anti-inflammatory drugs may be prescribed to relieve the pain and reduce inflammation. Corticosteroid injections to the shoulder may be used and physiotherapy may be required. Surgery is rarely used but is an option should all other treatments be unsuccessful.

Prognosis: Recovery can be slow - even taking several years - but most regain full movement.

Holistic Advice: It is important to keep as much movement as possible in the shoulder. Acupuncture claims to be effective in some cases. Bowen may possibly bring relief for some too.

Gallstones

Definition: Small stones that form in the gall bladder.

Possible Causes: It is thought that gallstones develop due to an imbalance in the chemical composition of bile. Gallstones are commonly made up of cholesterol and so a diet high in cholesterol may be a cause. Risk factors include age, sex (women are more likely to develop stones), obesity, cirrhosis and family history.

General Signs and Symptoms: Gallstones are present in about 1 in 10 people but usually go unnoticed. This is called asymptomatic gallstones. However, sudden and intense pain in the abdomen, nausea, vomiting and sweating (a collection of symptoms called biliary colic) may be experienced if stones become trapped and block a duct. This is called uncomplicated gallstones and usually lasts 1-5 hours. Complicated gallstones is the most serious, and occurs when the gallstones cause inflammation of the gall bladder, bile ducts or pancreas. These inflammatory conditions are associated with a high temperature and symptoms that last more than 8 hours. Complicated gallstones can be very serious and medical advice should be sought without delay.

Conventional Medical Treatment: The most effective treatment is to remove the gall bladder, but in mild cases the symptoms may not recur frequently and so surgery may not be necessary. Reducing the amount of fat in the diet may help and painkillers can be used during an attack. Less effective treatments include removing the gallstones but not the gall bladder, using drugs to dissolve the gallstones (if they are made of cholesterol) and using ultrasonic shock waves to break up the stones.

Prognosis: Removal of the gall bladder usually cures the problem. If the gall bladder is not removed there is an ongoing risk of recurrent attacks or gallstones reforming.

Holistic Advice: Eat a low fat, high fibre diet, lose any excess weight and take regular exercise.

Ganglion

Definition: A fluid-filled cyst that develops around joints and tendons.

Possible Causes: Arise when synovial fluid collects and forms a swelling. The exact cause is unknown but risk factors include ageing and injury.

General Signs and Symptoms: Smooth, soft lump under the skin. They commonly appear on the wrist, hand and fingers, but can occur around any joint or tendon in the body. They do not tend to cause pain, but a ganglion can cause discomfort if it affects a nerve or gets particularly large.

Conventional Medical Treatment: Treatment is only usually necessary if the ganglion is causing pain or is unsightly. If this is the case, it can be removed by draining out the fluid with a needle or syringe or by surgery.

Prognosis: Harmless and may disappear without treatment.

Holistic Advice: The "old wives' tale" of hitting a ganglion with a heavy book to disperse its contents is not conventionally recommended!

Gangrene

Definition: Death of tissue in a particular area of the body. There are several types. Wet and dry are covered below.

Possible Causes: Dry gangrene is the most common. It is caused when the tissues become deprived of oxygen, possibly due to a blood clot. The tissue death is localised and does not spread from the affected site. Wet gangrene occurs when the oxygen supply to tissue is suddenly restricted by a wound (e.g. burn, frostbite, crush injury) and becomes infected with bacteria. The infection can spread to surrounding healthy tissues and can be fatal. Diabetics are susceptible to wet gangrene after suffering a foot injury. Risk factors for gangrene include conditions that reduce blood flow, diabetes and smoking.

General Signs and Symptoms: The feet and legs are most commonly affected. In dry gangrene the skin at the affected area turns pale and cold, before turning from red to brown and then to black. The affected part withers and eventually drops off. This may be quite painless. Wet gangrene is very painful. The affected area swells before the tissues start to decay. The skin colour changes from red to brown and to then to black, and the tissues produce a foul smelling pus. The infection may also cause a fever.

Conventional Medical Treatment: Immediate hospitalisation is often required. The treatment aims to remove the affected tissue, treat the infection and address any underlying condition. Surgery or maggot therapy may be used to remove the dead tissue. In cases of wet gangrene, an area of surrounding living tissue will also be removed to attempt to control the spread of the infection. Antibiotics are commonly used. A variety of surgical techniques can be used to assist blood flow.

Prognosis: Potentially a life-threatening condition. The earlier it is diagnosed the better. If dry gangrene is caught early, the outlook is good. The outlook for wet gangrene is not so good due to the possible complications, including sepsis, caused by the infection.

Holistic Advice: Take regular exercise, stop smoking, ensure that the feet are well looked after, eat a well balanced diet, and lose any excess weight.

Gastritis

Definition: A common condition where the lining of the stomach becomes inflamed after damage.

Possible Causes: There are a wide range of common causes, including: infection by H. pylori bacteria, excessive alcohol or cocaine use, smoking, regular use of anti-inflammatory medication, injury, critical illness or major surgery. Less commonly, gastritis can be caused by an autoimmune reaction where the body attacks the stomach lining.

General Signs and Symptoms: Symptoms may come on suddenly (acutely) or over time (chronic). Gastritis can cause indigestion, stomach pain, feeling and being sick and feeling full after eating. In erosive gastritis the stomach lining will wear away leading to pain, bleeding and stomach ulcers. When caused by a bacterial infection there are often no symptoms.

Conventional Medical Treatment: The main aim of treatment is to reduce stomach acids to allow the stomach lining to heal. Antacids (to neutralise stomach acids), histamine 2 blockers (to decrease stomach acid production) and proton pump inhibitors such as omeprazole (to decrease stomach acid production) may be used to ease symptoms. If suspected cause is anti-inflammatory medication then a different medication will be tried. If gastritis is caused by the H.pylori bacteria then antibiotics as well as a proton pump inhibitor will be prescribed.

Prognosis: H.pylori stomach infection is usually lifelong so managing symptoms will be required. Chronic gastritis caused by other means can increase the risk of stomach ulcer, polyps (growths) in the stomach and stomach tumours (benign or malignant).

Holistic Advice: Avoid foods that may irritate the stomach (spicy, acidic, fried), reduce or eliminate alcohol consumption, eat little and often and stop smoking.

Gastroenteritis

Definition: Inflammation of the lining of the stomach and intestines.

Possible Causes: Usually caused by either a viral infection (e.g. norovirus) or a bacterial infection (e.g. E.coli and salmonella). Bacterial infections are often picked up from contaminated food or water, and there is an increased risk of this when travelling abroad. Most forms of gastroenteritis are highly infectious and are passed from stools to mouth when hygiene is poor.

General Signs and Symptoms: Symptoms rapidly develop and include diarrhoea, nausea, vomiting, stomach cramps and abdominal pain, fever and headache. The vomiting and diarrhoea can lead to dehydration. Symptoms of viral gastroenteritis tend to last 2-3 days, and bacterial gastroenteritis lasts 4-7 days.

Conventional Medical Treatment: Mild attacks usually clear up without treatment. Drink plenty of water to help avoid dehydration. Rehydration drinks can help rebalance the salt and sugar levels. Antidiarrhoeal drugs can help the diarrhoea but may prolong the presence of the infection. Anti-emetics can help reduce the vomiting. Antibiotics only tend to be prescribed in severe cases when a specific bacterium has been identified as the cause of the infection.

Prognosis: Usually harmless but the diarrhoea and vomiting can lead to dehydration, which can be serious for the very young and the elderly.

Holistic Advice: The risk of developing infectious gastroenteritis can be reduced by washing the hands regularly, particularly after going to the toilet and before eating. Practice good food hygiene to help prevent food poisoning and follow the recommended guidelines for safe eating and drinking when travelling abroad.

Genital Herpes

Definition: A viral infection that causes painful blisters on and around the genitals. It affects both men and women.

Possible Causes: Caused by the highly contagious herpes simplex virus (HSV). It is passed through skin-to-skin contact usually during sexual intercourse. There are two types of HSV, type 1 and type 2. Genital herpes is usually caused by type 2 HSV. Type 1 mainly causes cold sores on the mouth but can be transmitted from the mouth to the genitals where it may cause genital herpes. Once infected the virus can remain dormant within the nerves of the skin until an outbreak is triggered. Triggers may include illness, being run-down, stress and excess alcohol consumption. The changes in hormones during the menstrual cycle may trigger an outbreak in infected women.

General Signs and Symptoms: Symptoms may not appear for months even years after infection. If symptoms are to show soon after infection they usually do so within 4-7 days. Symptoms include painful, fluid-filled blisters on the genitals, thighs and buttocks that burst to leave ulcers, tingling burning and redness in the affected areas, pain on passing urine, headache, fever and muscle aches. Women may experience vaginal discharge and cervical blistering and ulceration. The first attack usually displays the worst symptoms. Recurrent infections tend to be shorter and less severe.

Conventional Medical Treatment: Anti-viral medicines (e.g. acyclovir) can be used to prevent the virus from multiplying, although it does not clear it from the body. Clinics specializing in sexually transmitted diseases (STDs) will be able to offer specialist help, advice and counselling. A pregnant women who has an attack just before childbirth may require a caesarean section to prevent infecting the baby. Painkillers and ointments for the blisters may help to relieve the symptoms.

Prognosis: There is no cure but the symptoms can generally be controlled by treatment. Genital herpes is often a chronic condition with frequent recurrences that decrease over time.

Holistic Advice: Prevention is better than (no) cure! Always practice safe sex. Although using a condom does not always prevent infection (due to contact with other parts of the skin that may be infected) it will reduce the risk. Avoid having sex during an outbreak when the virus is very contagious. It is advised that you do not share towels or flannels with your partner.

Gigantism

Definition: A rare condition where the body produces too much growth hormone before the end of puberty, when the epiphyseal growth plates of the long bones are still open. Gigantism is called acromegaly when it develops in adulthood.

Possible Causes: Gigantism occurs when the pituitary gland produces too much growth hormone. This is usually caused by a non-cancerous tumour (adenoma) on the pituitary gland.

General Signs and Symptoms: The most common symptom in young people is that they are abnormally tall in comparison to those of a similar age. They may also have very large hands/feet and large prominent facial features. If the adenoma is large and pushing on surrounding nerves then vision disturbances and headaches may be experienced. Puberty may be delayed and girls can experience an irregular menstrual cycle.

Conventional Medical Treatment: Treatment dependent on symptoms. The main aim is to reduce the production of growth hormone to normal levels. This is usually achieved via surgery to remove the tumour. In some instances the level of growth hormone may still be elevated, even after surgery. If this is the case injections of medication to slow the release or the effects of growth hormone will be used. If surgery and medication hasn't been totally effective then radiotherapy can be used to target the tumour.

Prognosis: Gigantism can be successfully treated but early diagnosis is key to reducing symptoms and preventing any further complications.

Holistic Advice: Maintain a healthy balanced diet for wellbeing.

Gingivitis

Definition: A common condition where the gums become swollen, sore or infected. Also known as mild gum disease.

Possible Causes: The most common cause of gingivitis is poor oral hygiene. This can be a result of not brushing the teeth regularly or properly allowing plaque to build on the teeth. The acid in plaque begins to break down the surface of the tooth and over time causes decay. Resulting bacteria can irritate the gums causing soreness and inflammation. The risk of developing issues with the gums increases if you smoke, have diabetes, are pregnant, have a weakened immune system, are malnourished or are under prolonged stress. Some medicines, such as antihistamines and antidepressants can cause a dry mouth can also increase the likeliness of developing gum disease.

General Signs and Symptoms: Early symptoms of gum disease, or gingivitis, include red, swollen gums and bleeding after brushing or flossing the teeth. This is not always painful and people are often unaware that they have it.

Conventional Medical Treatment: Practising good oral hygiene at home is the best way to treat and prevent gingivitis. Brush teeth for 2 minutes a time, twice a day. Daily usage of a good fluoride toothpaste will help protect against tooth decay. Regularly floss the teeth or use interdental brushes before brushing the teeth. A professional clean by a dental hygienist may be recommended if you are showing signs of gum disease.

Prognosis: Gingivitis can be effectively treated at home by practising good oral hygiene. If the plaque or tartar developed from gingivitis is not removed the condition could lead to periodontitis (gum disease). Periodontitis, if left untreated, can affect the tissues that support the teeth causing gum abscesses, receding gums and tooth loss.

Holistic Advice: Practice good oral hygiene. Do not smoke. Visit a dentist every 1 to 2 years for a check-up.

Glandular Fever

Definition: A viral infection causing swollen lymph nodes, a sore throat and fatigue. Also called infectious mononucleosis.

Possible Causes: Most cases are caused by the Epstein-Barr virus (EBV). The virus attacks lymphocytes that are responsible for fighting infection. The lymphocytes pass the infection on to the lymph nodes, spleen and liver. Most EBV infections take place during childhood with few symptoms, but when it occurs during the teenage or adult years it may lead to full blown glandular fever. Glandular fever is contagious and is commonly spread through saliva. Once in the body the EBV virus remains there for life. Other far less common causes of the condition include the cytomegalovirus and rubella.

General Signs and Symptoms: Swollen lymph glands particularly in the neck, armpits and groin, very sore throat, fatigue, fever, tonsillitis, headache, swollen spleen, tender abdomen, skin rash and loss of appetite. Infections affecting the liver may cause jaundice and hepatitis.

Conventional Medical Treatment: There is no cure. Rest, drinking plenty of water, and taking painkillers such as paracetamol may help ease the symptoms. Gargling with salt water may help the sore throat. Antibiotics may be used to treat secondary infections only.

Prognosis: Most symptoms usually pass within 4-6 weeks. The associated fatigue can last for longer. Complications are uncommon but serious, including a ruptured spleen or a secondary infection of the lungs.

Holistic Advice: Anything that can help boost the immune system will help the condition. Remember that glandular fever is contagious, and contagious diseases are usually contraindicated to hands-on complementary healthcare therapies.

Glomerulonephritis

Definition: Inflammation of the glomeruli (the filtering units) of the kidneys. Note, nephritis literally means inflammation (-itis) of the kidney (nephr-). There are 2 main types, primary, where the condition occurs on its own, and secondary, where the inflammation occurs as a result of an underlying condition. Glomerulonephritis can be acute or chronic.

Possible Causes: The inflammation affects kidney function. Salt and excess fluid can build up in the body and kidney damage or even kidney failure can occur. The cause is not always known, but it may be a complication arising from infection. It is thought the body's antibodies (produced to fight the antigens that create the infection) and the antigens themselves, build up in the kidneys, causing them to become inflamed. For example, acute glomerulonephritis can develop after infection by the streptococci bacteria, which causes throat infections. It can also be a complication of more serious infections such as HIV, hepatitis B and C, and tuberculosis. Risk factors include having an autoimmune condition such as lupus, some types of glomerulonephritis run in families, long term use of certain medications, and conditions that damage the kidneys such as cancer, leukaemia, diabetes, hypertension and liver disease.

General Signs and Symptoms: Blood and protein are passed in the urine. These may only be visibly noticeable when the kidneys have been severely damaged and so, in acute cases, may show up only in a urine test. In severe cases blood may be seen in the urine and the urine may appear cloudy or frothy. Other symptoms include the inability to urinate for 2-3 days, swollen feet and legs, puffy face, shortness of breath, headache, loss of appetite, vomiting, fever, pale skin and visual problems.

Conventional Medical Treatment: Treatment will depend on the cause and severity of the condition. In cases of bacterial infection, antibiotics may be used. If it is thought to be caused by an autoimmune disorder, immunosuppressant medication may be prescribed. Corticosteroids may be used to help reduce the inflammation. Diet and fluid intake will be regulated.

Prognosis: Acute cases tend to clear in 6-8 weeks. In some cases kidney function is reduced but does not deteriorate further, but others may develop chronic kidney failure. Hypertension, kidney disease and kidney failure are all known complications.

Holistic Advice: Reduce the amount of salt in the diet and drink less alcohol.

Goitre

Definition: Swelling of the thyroid gland causing a lump in the front of the neck. There are two main types, diffuse goitre and nodular goitre.

Possible Causes: A goitre can be caused by harmless nodules/cysts, dietary deficiencies (e.g lack of iodine), medications (e.g. lithium) and cancer treatments (e.g. radiotherapy). Hyperthyroidism, hypothyroidism, thyroid cancer and thyroiditis can cause a goitre to form. Hormone changes during puberty, pregnancy and the menopause can also be a cause. The risk of developing goitre increases with age and it is more common in women than men.

General Signs and Symptoms: Symptoms dependent on the size of the goitre, which can vary from person to person. Small swellings often do not cause symptoms. In severe cases coughing, tightness in the throat, changes to the voice, difficulty swallowing and difficulty breathing can be developed.

Conventional Medical Treatment: Treatment dependent on underlying cause, the size and the symptoms it is causing. For small goitre, which is causing little or no symptoms, a 'wait and see' approach may be taken. If caused by iodine deficiency, iodine supplements will be recommended. A type of radiotherapy called radioiodine treatment to destroy the thyroid cells and limit hormone production can be used for overactive thyroid. Surgery, or a thyroidectomy, to remove all or part of the thyroid is performed when breathing or swallowing is compromised and other forms of treatment have not been successful.

Prognosis: Dependent on the underlying cause. If the thyroid is removed then medication will need to be taken to replicate normal thyroid function. Thyroid surgery can have complications such as infection, nerve damage and damage to the parathyroid gland that sits behind the thyroid.

Holistic Advice: Maintain a healthy balanced diet for wellbeing. Include white fish, shellfish, dairy and sea vegetables (seaweed) as a source of iodine if required.

Gonorrhoea

Definition: A sexually transmitted infection caused by bacteria.

Possible Causes: Caused by Neisseria gonorrhoeae or gonococcus bacteria which is mainly found in fluids from the penis or vagina. It is spread via unprotected sexual intercourse or the sharing of sex toys. Pregnant women with gonorrhoea can pass it onto their baby during childbirth.

General Signs and Symptoms: Symptoms usually develop within 2 weeks of being infected. In women, unusual vaginal discharge (thin/watery and green or yellow in colour), pain or burning when urinating are most common. Infrequently, pain in the lower abdomen and bleeding in between periods or after sex occur. In men, unusual discharge from the tip of the penis (white, yellow or green in colour), pain or burning when urinating and inflammation of the foreskin are all common. Pain or tenderness in the testicles can also occur but is uncommon. Both men and women can develop infections in the rectum, throat and eyes if infected semen or vaginal fluid comes into contact with these areas. When passed from Mother to baby during childbirth the baby will develop red and swollen eyes with a pus-like discharge.

Conventional Medical Treatment: Prevention is better than cure. Most commonly treated with a short course of antibiotics. A follow up test will be scheduled to ensure the infection has gone. It is also safe to give babies antibiotics and these will be administered immediately after birth. Current and recent sexual partners should also be tested and treated.

Prognosis: If treated early it is very unlikely to cause any issues. Without treatment it can spread to other parts of the body and cause serious complications. In women, gonorrhoea can spread through the reproductive system causing pelvic inflammatory disease. During pregnancy the bacteria can cause miscarriage and premature labour. In men, gonorrhoea can cause painful infections in the testicles and prostate gland. Although rare, the bacteria can spread into the bloodstream and cause sepsis.

Holistic Advice: Prevention is key; use of a condom or barrier during sexual intercourse. Avoid sharing sex toys, if you do share them ensure they are covered with a condom and cleaned after use.

Gout

Definition: Gout, a common type of arthritis, is an intermittent constitutional disorder affecting small joints.

Possible Causes: Excess uric acid (a waste product of metabolism) in the blood causes crystals to form in the joints. Excess uric acid is caused either because too much is being produced or because it is not being excreted adequately by the kidneys. The excessive intake of food rich in purines is a significant risk factor. Purines are a type of acid that are found in foods such as red meats and seafood, and are also present in alcohol (especially beer). Gout can be familial and some medical conditions such as hypertension, psoriasis, diabetes, kidney problems, and high cholesterol levels can increase the risk of it developing. Some medications can also increase uric acid levels and so increase the likelihood of gout.

General Signs and Symptoms: Pain and inflammation of a joint, normally the big toe. The skin over the affected area may appear red and shiny, and may become itchy and flaky. Gout is more predominant in males over forty years old. It can attack quickly and without warning, often during the night.

Conventional Medical Treatment: Anti-inflammatory drugs are used to reduce the inflammation and the pain or, in more severe cases, corticosteroids. To prevent further attacks, drugs can be prescribed to reduce uric acid levels. Lifestyle changes to control diet, reduce alcohol intake, increase water intake, and avoid excessive weight gain are very important.

Prognosis: Gout can disappear on its own within 3-10 days. A combination of medical treatment and lifestyle changes can enable uric acid levels to be reduced, and so help prevent further attacks.

Holistic Advice: Look at diet. Avoid purine-high foods and alcohol. Try to avoid knocking the affected joint, elevate it, and keep it cool. Drink plenty of water. Uric acid levels are often higher in those who are overweight, so try to lose excess weight.

Graves' Disease

Definition: An autoimmune disease where the immune system attacks the thyroid gland, causing it to make too much thyroid hormone. A common cause of hyperthyroidism.

Possible Causes: Exact cause is unknown. Those commonly affected are young to middle aged women, particularly if Graves' disease runs in the family. Smoking is thought to be a risk factor.

General Signs and Symptoms: Symptoms are those of hyperthyroidism, for example hyperactivity, weight loss, rapid heartbeat, hand tremors, excessive sweating, intolerance to heat, anxiety, insomnia, frequent bowel movements, swelling in the neck caused by an enlarged thyroid (goitre), loss of libido and muscle weakness. A more specific symptom of Graves' disease is bulging eyes and skin thickening, particularly over the lower legs and feet.

Conventional Medical Treatment: Treatment aims to reduce the amount of thyroid hormones produced. Options include anti-thyroid drugs, to suppress the production of the thyroid hormones, radioactive iodine, to destroy part of the thyroid, and surgical removal of a part of the thyroid or all of it (less common in Graves' Disease). Betablockers may be prescribed to counter some of the symptoms such as the hyperactivity, rapid heartbeat and tremors.

Prognosis: Most fully recover. Some treatments may result in the thyroid producing too little thyroid hormones and so hormone supplements may be required. In very rare cases, failure to treat an overactive thyroid may result in a thyroid storm. This serious condition requires urgent medical attention.

Holistic Advice: Stop smoking. Thyroid hormone levels should be monitored regularly after treatment.

Haematoma

Definition: An abnormal collection of blood outside a blood vessel. Haematomas are described based on their location.

Possible Causes: When a blood vessel is damaged, blood will leak into the surrounding tissue and pool. The greater the bleeding, the larger the haematoma. Trauma is the most common cause. Trauma can range from severe, like a car accident or fall, to mild, like a powerful sneeze or unexpected twist of a leg. Viral infection such as rubella, mumps HIV and hepatitis C are also associated with haematomas. Certain blood thinning medications including warfarin and aspirin can increase the chance of spontaneous bleeding. People at a higher risk of developing haematoma include those with blood cancer, chronic liver disease and bleeding disorders such as haemophilia. Serious conditions such as an aneurysm also cause large haematomas.

General Signs and Symptoms: Symptoms often depend on the location of the haematoma but they often cause irritation and inflammation in the surrounding area/structures bringing redness, warmth, swelling and pain. Haematoma occurring in the brain (epidural and subdural haematoma) is very serious, causing severe headache, confusion, nausea, vomiting, seizures, slurred speech and loss of consciousness.

Conventional Medical Treatment: Treatment depends on the location and size of the haematoma. Some may require no treatment and others may be a medical emergency. Haematoma in the soft tissue, like the muscle, can be treated with rest, ice, compression and elevation (RICE). Surgical drainage is a common treatment for haematoma in the brain (subdural haematoma) and under the finger or toenail (subungual haematoma) if it is causing troublesome symptoms.

Prognosis: Overall haematomas resolve by themselves and do not cause any lasting damage. Haematomas occurring the brain are a medical emergency and can result in death.

Holistic Advice: Try to rest the affected area if possible. Seek medical treatment immediately for severe head injuries or minor head injuries where the above symptoms occur.

Haemophilia

Definition: A rare condition that affects blood clotting.

Possible Causes: Caused by an inherited genetic mutation on the X chromosome which can be passed to a child from their Mother, Father or both. The mutation affects the clotting factors in the blood by reducing the amount present. The majority of people who have it are male and there are cases where boys are born with the condition and no family history. The chances of the gene being inherited by the child depends on which of their parents have the gene.

General Signs and Symptoms: Dependent on the severity and the amount of clotting factors present in the blood. The main sign is prolonged bleeding which can happen spontaneously. Those with mild haemophilia may not see symptoms unless they have a wound, surgery or invasive dental procedure where they might experience a long period of bleeding. Moderate haemophiliacs may have additional symptoms such as internal bleeding around the joints. This is most commonly experienced around the ankles, knees and elbows. In severe haemophilia, in addition to the above, there is high risk of spontaneous bleeding in the form of nosebleeds, joints bleeds, muscles bleeds and bleeding gums.

Conventional Medical Treatment: Treatment plans depend on severity of the condition. In mild – moderate cases, treatment may be administered on-demand and in response to bleeding. This will be in form of injections. In severe haemophilia, preventative treatment involves regular injections of medication to increase the specific clotting factors needed in the blood.

Prognosis: There is no cure for haemophilia however treatment and management allows the individual to have a good quality of life. Preventative treatment is often continued for life but some people are able to move to on-demand treatment. It is possible for the immune system to develop antibodies, called inhibitors, against the treatment injections. Joint damage from bleeding is a common complication for older adults with severe haemophilia though it is hoped that modern treatments will help younger people with haemophilia today.

Holistic Advice: Avoid contact sports. Avoid medicines that affect the bloods ability to clot (aspirin). Have regular dental appointments and take good care of the teeth and gums.

Haemorrhoids

Definition: Swollen veins inside the rectum and around the anus. Commonly called piles. There are two main types; internal (occurring inside the rectum) and external (occurring outside the rectum). Internal are more common.

Possible Causes: An increase in pressure on the blood vessels causes them to swell. This is usually as a result of straining when passing a stool. Risk factors include obesity, constipation, low-fibre diet, prolonged diarrhoea, heavy lifting, pregnancy, age and family history.

General Signs and Symptoms: Discomfort when passing a stool, bleeding from the anus after a bowel movement, discharge of mucus after a bowel movement, itchy and sore anus, and feeling that the bowels have not fully emptied. Haemorrhoids may be seen protruding from the anus. These are called prolapsed haemorrhoids.

Conventional Medical Treatment: Small haemorrhoids do not usually require treatment and clear up of their own accord. Over-the-counter creams, ointments and suppositories are available to help the itching and pain. Topical corticosteroids may be prescribed. Laxatives may ease the passing of stools in cases where the haemorrhoids are caused by constipation. Several surgical options are available, including banding (to shrink the haemorrhoid until it eventually drops off), injections (to relieve pain and destroy the haemorrhoid), infrared coagulation (to destroy the haemorrhoid using heat), or their complete surgical removal.

Prognosis: Not usually serious.

Holistic Advice: Eat a high-fibre diet. Any bleeding from the anus should be investigated by a Doctor, because it can also be indicative of a more serious disorder.

Hashimoto's Thyroiditis

Definition: Swelling of the thyroid gland specifically caused by the immune system.

Possible Causes: The thyroid is attacked by the immune system, which over time makes the thyroid unable to produce enough thyroid hormone. This in turn causes hypothyroidism (underactive thyroid). Much more common in women than in men, it is not clear what causes the immune system to attack the thyroid. It can take months or even years for this slow progressing disease to be detected.

General Signs and Symptoms: Due to the nature of the disease symptoms will progress slowly. Symptoms of an underactive thyroid include weight gain, muscle aches and extreme tiredness. Other early symptoms include cramps, sensitivity to cold, constipation, slowness in body and mind, muscle weakness, dry skin, brittle hair and nails, heavy or irregular periods and depression. A swollen thyroid may also cause a goitre (lump) to form in the throat.

Conventional Medical Treatment: Medication will be prescribed to rebalance the levels of thyroid hormone. The amount taken should be regularly monitored. Surgery is rare and only if the goitre is very uncomfortable or there is suspected cancer.

Prognosis: Hashimoto's thyroiditis cannot be cured and there is a high possibility that medication to keep the thyroid hormone levels stable will need to be taken for the rest of the person's life.

Holistic Advice: Exercise regularly and maintain a healthy balanced diet.

Hay Fever

Definition: Inflammation of the membrane lining the nose and throat due to an allergic reaction. Also called seasonal allergic rhinitis (inflammation of the nose).

Possible Causes: Allergic reaction to substances such as pollen or spores resulting in the inflammation of the nose, sinuses, throat and eyes. The presence of the allergen causes the cells to release histamine, which triggers the allergic reaction so causing the symptoms. Risk factors include family history or allergies, particularly asthma or eczema.

General Signs and Symptoms: Itchy eyes, throat, mouth, nose and ears, headache, violent sneezing, watery eyes and nose, and a dry cough. Usually occurs in the spring and summer when there is more pollen in the air. The severity of the hay fever depends on weather conditions and the pollen count.

Conventional Medical Treatment: Antihistamine tablets and nasal sprays help block the action of the histamine. Corticosteroid nasal spray and drops have an anti-inflammatory effect. Nasal decongestants can help blocked noses, and eye drops can help treat red, itchy eyes. Immunotherapy may be used.

Prognosis: There is no cure but the treatments can help to alleviate the symptoms. Hay fever can worsen respiratory conditions such as asthma.

Holistic Advice: Try to avoid the trigger. Avoid dairy products as these may cause additional mucus to form which can worsen the condition. Homeopathy, acupuncture and herbal remedies claim to be of benefit.

Headache (Tension)

Definition: Pain or discomfort, of variable intensity, in the head and neck.

Possible Causes: Most headaches have no underlying medical condition but are triggered by a range of factors such as stress, tension, depression, anxiety, loud noise, poor posture, bright sunlight, eyestrain, tiredness, certain foods, hunger, anger, hormonal changes, certain smells, changes in the weather and the long term use of painkillers. These are called primary headaches and include tension headaches, cluster headaches (very painful, short lived headaches that occur several times a day) and migraines (intense headache, often associated with visual disturbances and nausea). Secondary headaches are caused by an underlying condition such as meningitis and brain tumours. We'll focus on tension headaches here.

General Signs and Symptoms: Constant ache, affecting both sides of the head, tightening of neck muscles and a feeling of pressure behind the eyes. Normally comes on gradually and builds up during the day.

Conventional Medical Treatment: Over-the-counter painkillers (e.g. paracetamol) and anti-inflammatory drugs (e.g. ibuprofen) can usually relieve the pain.

Prognosis: Very common condition, generally successfully relieved by medication and changes in lifestyle.

Holistic Advice: Take measures to reduce stress, take regular exercise, practice relaxation techniques such as yoga and meditation, and reduce alcohol and caffeine intake. Medical advice should be sought if a severe headache does not respond to treatment and lasts for more than 24 hours.

Head Lice

Definition: A condition caused by the infestation of head louse (pediculus humanus capitis). Head lice infestation is also known as pediculosis capitis or nits.

Possible Causes: Infestation of the hair and scalp by head lice. These small insects are transferred from person to person by head-to-head contact.

General Signs and Symptoms: Itching on the head and the sensation of movement in the hair. Live lice will be present as well as eggs.

Conventional Medical Treatment: Treatment should start immediately following detection. Lice can be found and removed by using a fine toothed detection comb pulled through wet hair. If live lice are still being detected after 17 days, a pharmacist may advise medicated lotion to kill the lice.

Prognosis: Head lice cannot be prevented so stopping the spread is the best course of action. Treatment should eradicate the infestation within a few weeks.

Holistic Advice: Treat immediately following detection. Avoid so-called preventative treatments as these often irritate the scalp.

Heart Attack

Definition: Sudden loss of blood supply to part of the heart muscle. The medical term for this is myocardial infarction and it is also commonly called a coronary.

Possible Causes: Usually caused by coronary artery disease. This causes the coronary arteries to narrow due to atherosclerosis. Blood clots form in the narrowed arteries and if the artery blocks completely a heart attack results. Risk factors include smoking, obesity, lack of physical activity, high fat diet, family history of coronary heart disease, hypertension and diabetes.

General Signs and Symptoms: Sudden onset of severe, crushing pain in the centre of the chest. This may spread up to the neck and into the arms, especially the left arm. The skin becomes pale and there is sweating and shortness of breath. There may be nausea and vomiting. Great anxiety, sometimes accompanied by the fear of dying, is often experienced. Contrary to popular belief, heart attacks can occur without chest pain. Always take into account the whole picture. Should the blood supply not be restored quickly the heart muscle may suffer irreversible damage and the heart may stop beating. This is called a cardiac arrest.

Conventional Medical Treatment: The priority is to relieve pain and restore the blood supply to the heart muscle. Morphine may be used for the pain and medication such as thrombolytics (to reduce the clot) and anticoagulants (to help prevent further clots) may be used. There are several surgical procedures to aid blood flow to the heart, e.g. coronary artery bypass graft (to bypass the blockage) and angioplasty (to widen the artery at the site of the blockage). The treatment usually also requires lifestyle changes. Medication such as ACE inhibitors, beta-blockers, statins and anti-platelets may be prescribed to help reduce the risk of another heart attack.

Prognosis: All heart attacks are potentially life threatening. Just over half of those who have a heart attack die but, in cases where there is not a history of heart attacks, the prognosis is good if treated quickly and there are no complications.

Holistic Advice: Treat any suspected heart attack as a medical emergency. Post-heart attack the patient may be very fearful of returning to normal activity so consider the emotional state. Eat a low fat diet. Stop smoking and reduce alcohol intake. Take regular, gentle exercise. Try to tackle any sources of stress.

Heart Disease

Definition: Where fatty deposits narrow or block blood vessels around the heart. Also referred to as coronary heart disease, coronary artery disease and ischaemic heart disease.

Possible Causes: Narrowing or blocking of the blood vessels around the heart is caused by a build-up of fatty deposits called atheroma. This process is called atherosclerosis (see page 31). The risk of developing atherosclerosis is increased by smoking, sedentary lifestyle, being overweight or obese and a diet high in cholesterol and fat. Other risk factors include hypertension, diabetes and a family history of heart disease.

General Signs and Symptoms: Symptoms can vary between individuals and some may not experience symptoms prior to diagnosis. Angina (chest pain) and breathlessness are the most common symptoms. Shortness of breath, feeling faint and nausea may also be experienced. If the blood vessels become completely blocked it can cause a heart attack (myocardial infarction).

Conventional Medical Treatment: Treatment aims to manage symptoms and reduce risk of further complications. Lifestyle changes such as eating heathier and taking regular exercise are very important. Medication such as blood thinners, statins (to reduce cholesterol), beta-blockers or ACE inhibitors (to reduce blood pressure) and nitrates (to widen blood vessels) can be prescribed. Surgery may be recommended to open up or bypass blocked arteries. Coronary angioplasty and coronary artery bypass graft are the two most common options. On rare occasions a heart transplant may be performed if the heart is badly damaged and other treatment options haven't been effective.

Prognosis: With correct treatment, symptoms can be well managed and the function of the heart can be improved.

Holistic Advice: Stop smoking and reduce alcohol consumption. Eat a healthy balanced diet and take regular exercise. Maintain a healthy body weight.

Heart Failure

Definition: Where the heart is unable to pump blood around the body correctly.

Possible Causes: Usually a combination of problems affecting the heart at the same time, making the heart weak or stiff. Conditions such as coronary heart disease, high blood pressure, cardiomyopathy, heart rhythm issues and damage/problems with the heart valves can all lead to heart failure. People with birth defects from congenital heart disease are at risk of developing heart failure. In some cases anaemia, high pressure in the lungs (pulmonary hypertension) and hyperthyroidism can also lead to heart failure. Risk factors include excessive alcohol consumption and age.

General Signs and Symptoms: Symptoms vary from person to person and can come on suddenly or develop slowly over time. The most common symptoms are breathlessness (particularly at night when asleep), fatigue and swollen ankles and legs. Less common symptoms include persistent coughing, wheezing, dizziness, heart palpitations and a fast heart rate. Some people may notice a change in their weight and feel bloated and/or have a loss of appetite.

Conventional Medical Treatment: Treatment depends on severity, usually categorised by classes; class 1 being least severe and class 4 being most severe. Treatment often requires lifestyle changes. Combinations of medications are most commonly used to control the condition. These include medication to lower the blood pressure (ACE inhibitors and AR blockers), lower the heart rate (beta blockers) and remove swelling from the lower extremities (diuretics). In some cases devices will need to be implanted into the chest to control the rhythm of the heart (pacemaker, or implantable cardioverter defibrillator (ICD) or both). If the valves of the heart are affected, replacement or repair surgery may be required. Angioplasty or bypass could be recommended if the heart failure is related to coronary heart disease. A heart transplant is the last resort in very severe cases where other treatments fail.

Prognosis: Heart failure is a long-term condition that usually cannot be cured but can be managed. Regular reviews with the GP or care team will be required. Heart failure usually gets worse slowly over time and eventually will become severe.

Holistic Advice: Take medicines regularly as prescribed. Eat a healthy, balanced diet. Exercise regularly. Stop smoking and reduce alcohol consumption.

Heartburn

Definition: Regurgitation of acidic stomach juices into the oesophagus. Also called Gastro-oesophageal reflex disease (GORD).

Possible Causes: Sometimes there is no obvious cause for GORD. However, it can be caused by a malfunction of the lower oesophageal sphincter, which allows stomach acid to pass back into the oesophagus. Other causes are an increased pressure on the stomach causing the reflux, and stomach acid taking longer than usual to dispel. Risk factors include being overweight, a high fat diet, tobacco, alcohol, coffee, chocolate, stress, pregnancy and the presence of a hiatus hernia.

General Signs and Symptoms: A burning sensation rising from the stomach or lower chest into the throat, and regurgitation of acid into the throat or mouth. Sufferers may also belch. Symptoms are usually worse after a large meal, at night and when lying flat. Persistent GORD can cause permanent damage and scarring to the oesophageal lining. This can lead to complications such as oesophageal ulcers, oesophageal stricture and a condition called Barrett's oesophagus in which parts of the oesophageal lining is replaced by stomach lining. Sufferers of Barrett's oesophagus have an increased risk of oesophageal cancer.

Conventional Medical Treatment: Symptoms can be relieved by making lifestyle changes and antacids are usually successful in relieving mild symptoms. If the GORD persists, treatments may be used to reduce the amount of acid produced by the stomach or increase the speed at which the stomach empties.

Prognosis: Lifestyle changes can make a difference and treatments tend to be successful. Persistent GORD has complications as described above.

Holistic Advice: Eat smaller meals, do not exercise or lie down immediately after a meal, lose excess weight and stop smoking. Avoid spicy, acidic and high fat foods, carbonated drinks, alcohol and coffee. Look for triggers that make the GORD worse and then avoid them.

Heel Fissures

Definition: Cracked, split heels.

Possible Causes: The fissures (cracks) are usually caused by dry skin but other causes include inactive sweat glands, prolonged standing, obesity, foot problems including heel spurs and gait. Other skin conditions such as psoriasis and eczema may increase the chance of fissures.

General Signs and Symptoms: The fissures are usually in an area of dry, callused skin. Commonly they are only superficial but if they are deep they may cause bleeding and pain which is worsened by walking. Fissures may occur on other parts of the foot, particularly the bottom of the toes.

Conventional Medical Treatment: Heel fissures are usually a cosmetic problem, not a medical one, although treatment may be necessary in extreme cases if they become infected or if any of the hard skin needs to be removed by a Doctor or Chiropodist/Podiatrist. Special foot creams can be used to help this condition. The hard skin can be gradually removed by soaking the feet in warm water and then gently rubbing them with a pumice stone. A Podiatrist may recommend insoles to correct gait or heel-cups to support the heel.

Prognosis: No permanent damage should be caused.

Holistic Advice: Buy shoes with a good shock-absorbing sole and avoid those with open-backs. Keep the feet moisturised and try to avoid the formation of calluses.

Hepatitis

Description: Inflammation of the liver, usually caused by a virus. Sometimes, in mild cases, it is asymptomatic and the person may not even be aware that they are infected and successfully fight off the virus. In others, hepatitis can cause irreversible liver damage. The condition can be acute, causing discomfort in the upper right side of the abdomen, nausea, vomiting and a fever, or chronic, causing loss of appetite, weight loss, tiredness, jaundice, swelling of the abdomen and abdominal discomfort. Cirrhosis of the liver can be caused by long-term inflammation. There are several types of hepatitis including:

Hepatitis A: Caused by the hepatitis A virus. Most common in countries with poor sanitation and sewage. It is contracted from the stools of an infected person and can be passed to others in contaminated food or water. It is usually acute and vaccinations are available.

Hepatitis B: Caused by the hepatitis B virus. The virus lives in the body fluids (e.g. blood, saliva and semen) of an infected person and is passed from person to person by direct contact with these fluids, for example during sex or sharing contaminated intravenous needles. It can be transmitted from mother to baby. Many will not even know they are infected and will successfully fight the infection but, in some, it can develop into a chronic condition. There is a vaccine available.

Hepatitis C: Caused by the hepatitis C virus. The virus is mostly found in blood but can also be found in other body fluids. It is therefore predominantly passed by blood-to-blood contact, most commonly by sharing intravenous needles. Some can fight off the infection but others may develop a chronic illness resulting in cirrhosis of the liver, even liver failure. There is no vaccine. Some drugs are available that have been shown to clear the infection in about 50% of cases.

Noninfectious Hepatitis: Inflammation of the liver can also be caused by excessive alcohol consumption, other toxins (such as those found in some poisonous fungi), some drugs, and an overdose of paracetamol. There is also an autoimmune disease, called autoimmune hepatitis, in which the white blood cells attack the liver causing severe inflammation and liver damage.

Holistic Advice: Prevention is better than cure. Practice safe sex, maintain good hand hygiene and drink alcohol responsibly. Eat a healthy, balanced diet and take regular exercise to help keep the immune system in good shape.

__Hiatus Hernia__

Definition: The protrusion of a portion of the stomach through the diaphragm. The general term "hernia" is used to describe the protrusion of a part of an organ through a weakened muscle. "Hiatus" is the opening in the diaphragm through which the oesophagus passes. The hiatus is the weakened area through which the stomach protrudes in a hiatus hernia.

Possible Causes: Exact cause is unknown but it may be caused by pressure on the abdomen (e.g. sudden exertion, straining, coughing and being obese), a weakened diaphragm or a congenital defect of the diaphragm. Risk factors include being female, being over 50, pregnancy, being overweight and smoking.

General Signs and Symptoms: Can be asymptomatic. However, the protrusion of the stomach through the diaphragm can prevent the sphincter at the top of the stomach from working effectively. This may allow stomach contents to pass back up into the oesophagus causing heartburn, gastro-oesophageal reflux, deep burning chest pain and difficultly swallowing.

Conventional Medical Treatment: When no symptoms are present, no treatment is required. Antacids and a change of lifestyle are recommended to begin with. A variety of drugs to counter the impact of the ineffective sphincter are available. If medication is not successful, corrective surgery can be used to return the stomach to its correct location.

Prognosis: Not usually serious but persistent acid reflux can damage the oesophagus, increasing the risk of oesophageal cancer. Rarely the hernia may become strangulated, cutting off the blood supply. This requires emergency surgery.

Holistic Advice: Lose excess weight and stop smoking. Always use correct lifting techniques when moving heavy weights.

Hiccups

Definition: Sudden involuntary contractions of the diaphragm that cause the vocal to close, resulting in a 'hic' sound. Also known as hiccoughs.

Possible Causes: There is often no reason as to why hiccups start. Some commonly reported triggers are stress, certain medications, strong emotions such as excitement, laughing too much, eating or drinking too quickly (particularly fizzy drinks).

General Signs and Symptoms: Hiccups can occur singularly or in a series. Often a brief unexpected tremor affecting the shoulders, abdomen, throat or full body will occur, followed by an audible 'hic' or 'chirp' as the vocal cords shut.

Conventional Medical Treatment: A bout of hiccups is usually 'waited out' as in the large majority of cases they will cease by themselves. If hiccups last longer than 48 hours, seek medical advice.

Prognosis: Should stop eventually after a short period. If hiccups are prolonged (over 48 hours) or occur so regularly they are a disruption to daily life, a GP may look for underlying health conditions. If there is no obvious cause, chlorpromazine may be prescribed.

Holistic Advice: Sip ice cold water, bite on a lemon, swallow a small amount of granulated sugar, hold your breath for a short time or breathe into a paper bag (do not put the bag over your head).

High Cholesterol

Definition: Raised level of cholesterol in the blood. Called hypercholesterolaemia.

Possible Causes: Cholesterol is a lipid. It is transported around the body in the form of two types of lipoproteins, low-density (LDL) and high density (HDL). Too much LDL can cause a build up of deposits on the artery walls and so is known as "bad" cholesterol. HDL helps to carry the cholesterol back to the liver and is therefore referred to as "good" cholesterol. Blood tests are used to measure the cholesterol level and the government recommends that cholesterol levels should be less than 5mmol/L. High cholesterol levels are believed to be caused by a combination of genetic and lifestyle factors. A diet high in saturated fats, being overweight and a lack of exercise are thought to contribute. Other risk factors include smoking, diabetes, hypertension, hypothyroidism, excessive alcohol consumption, age, ethnicity, and a family history of cardiovascular disease or high cholesterol levels.

General Signs and Symptoms: High cholesterol is not a disease in itself but does increase the risk of serious cardiovascular conditions. A high cholesterol level usually goes unnoticed until it leads to the development of a disorder such as atherosclerosis. The symptoms will then be dependent on the location of the arterial narrowing.

Conventional Medical Treatment: A diet low in saturated fat can reduce levels of LDL. For those with high risk factors, making it more likely that the high cholesterol level will cause cardiovascular diseases, a change in diet is not sufficient to lower the risk, and so medication will usually be prescribed. The most common type of medication to lower cholesterol levels is statins. Other medication can be given to help reduce the risk of associated strokes and heart attacks (e.g. aspirin to help prevent blood clotting).

Prognosis: Medication and lifestyle changes tend to be successful in bringing down cholesterol levels. The extent of the risk of having a high cholesterol level depends upon the presence of risk factors. It is widely accepted that a high cholesterol level increases the risk of cardiovascular disease.

Holistic Advice: Medication and lifestyle changes tend to be successful in bringing down cholesterol levels. The extent of the risk of having a high cholesterol level depends upon the presence of risk factors. It is widely accepted that a high cholesterol level increases the risk of cardiovascular disease.

Hirsutism

Definition: Abnormal and excessive hair growth, indicating underlying hormonal issues in women.

Possible Causes: An increase in the amount and/or the body's sensitivity to androgens (often referred to as 'male' hormones). Polycystic ovary syndrome (PCOS) is the most common cause. On rare occasions, other hormonal conditions such as Cushing's syndrome and acromegaly as well as certain medications and anabolic steroids can cause hirsutism. Being overweight or having a family of the condition increases the risk of it developing.

General Signs and Symptoms: Excessive thick dark hair growth on the face and body including the neck, chest, tummy, lower back, buttocks and thighs.

Conventional Medical Treatment: The hair growth only requires treatment if is bothersome to the individual. Home hair lightening and removal treatments can be used. Prescription creams can be used to slow hair growth on the face. Electrolysis and laser hair removal may be recommended for longer-term hair removal. Weight loss (if overweight) and taking the contraceptive pill can help control hormone levels.

Prognosis: The hair growth itself will not cause any long-term complications, however it can be detrimental to the mental health of the individual. Underlying hormone imbalances can be indicative of other conditions.

Holistic Advice: Maintain a healthy weight.

HIV and AIDS

Definition: A long term infection which, if left untreated, results in reduced immunity to other infections.

Possible Causes: The condition is caused by the Human Immunodeficiency Virus (HIV). HIV is spread by the exchange of body fluids including blood, semen, vaginal or anal secretions and breast milk. Transmission commonly takes place during sexual intercourse, the sharing of needles and during pregnancy, when the foetus becomes infected via vascular connections with the mother. HIV attacks the immune system leaving the sufferer with a high risk of developing a serious infection or disease. AIDS (Acquired Immune Deficiency Syndrome) occurs when the HIV infection renders the immune system inactive and the sufferer develops a life-threatening condition such as pneumonia. AIDS now tends to be referred to as advanced or late-stage HIV infection.

General Signs and Symptoms: The initial signs of HIV infection include a fever, sore throat, tiredness, joint and muscle pain, swollen glands and a blotchy rash on the chest. After the initial symptoms, HIV may not display any symptoms for many years but will be progressively damaging the immune system. Left untreated the infection may cause a range of late-stage symptoms including persistent tiredness, night sweats, weight loss, diarrhoea, blurred vision, white spots on the tongue or mouth, dry cough, shortness of breath, fever and swollen glands. AIDS-related illnesses such as tuberculosis, pneumonia, nervous system disorders and some cancers may be caused.

Conventional Medical Treatment: There is no cure and no vaccine to stop infection, but treatments can help control the HIV infection so holding off AIDS. Antiretroviral therapy (ART) is often successful in slowing the progression of the disease with the goal of an undetectable viral load i.e. the level of HIV virus in the blood is so low it is undetectable, therefore preventing transmission. Post Exposure Prophylaxis (PEP) may possibly halt the development of HIV if used within 72 hours of exposure to the virus.

Prognosis: The advances in treatment have transformed the prognosis from rapidly fatal condition to a long-term illness.

Holistic Advice: Prevention is the best cure. Using condoms correctly prevents contact with semen or vaginal secretions. It may be beneficial for HIV positive individuals to make those who treat them (e.g. health care professionals or dentists) aware of the infection so they can they can provide appropriate medication and care. Anything to boost the immune system may be of benefit. Emotional support and practical advice can be obtained through help groups.

Hodgkin Lymphoma

Definition: An uncommon cancer that develops in the lymphatic system.

Possible Causes: A mutation in white blood cells, specifically B-lymphocytes. This mutation causes the B-lymphocytes to multiply uncontrollably. Slightly more common in women, it is not clear what triggers or causes this to happen. Risk factors that increase the chance of developing this condition include a weakened immune system from conditions such as HIV, taking immunosuppressant drugs, previous exposure to the Epstein-Barr virus that causes glandular fever, previous incidence of non-Hodgkin lymphoma and being obese.

General Signs and Symptoms: The most common symptom are painless swellings in the neck, armpit or groin. This is caused by excess B-lymphocytes collecting in the lymph nodes. Symptoms can be location specific such as abdominal pain if the abdomen is affected. Sometimes there will be more generalised symptoms such as night sweats, unexpected weight loss, fever, persistent cough and an itching sensation over the skin.

Conventional Medical Treatment: The main treatment is chemotherapy. This may be paired with radiotherapy or steroid medication. In rare cases a biological therapies are used in combination with chemotherapy.

Prognosis: Overall, treatment is highly effective and most go into remission. Some people will experience long term problems including a weakened immune system, infertility and secondary cancers such as lymphoma and leukaemia. The risk of developing cardiovascular and lung disease increases after having Hodgkin Lymphoma.

Holistic Advice: Maintain a healthy weight. Take steps to boost the immune system.

Hydronephrosis

Definition: The stretching or swelling of one or both kidneys.

Possible Causes: The most common cause is a blockage in the urinary system. The blockage can be in ureters, the point at which the renal pelvis of the kidney joins the ureter, in the bladder or in the urethra. Blockages in the ureters affect just one kidney (unilateral hydronephrosis) but blockages in the bladder and urethra affect them both (bilateral hydronephrosis). Narrowing or blocking of the ureters can be caused by many factors including an abnormality that is present at birth, a kidney stone in the ureter, growths, tumours, narrowing resulting from injury, infection, constriction, surgery, or a disorder of the nerves and muscles in the ureter. Bladder blockages can be caused by a bladder stone, blood clot, tumour, inflammation or having pressure exerted upon it (e.g. as in prostatitis). Urethral blockages can be caused by strictures and pressure. Bilateral hydronephrosis can also be caused by the backflow of urine from the bladder to the kidneys. This is usually due to a malfunction of the one-way valve in the bladder.

General Signs and Symptoms: The symptoms will depend on the location of the blockage, whether it suddenly or progressively develops, the length of time the flow of urine is interrupted, and the extent that the kidney(s) is stretched. When a blockage occurs suddenly, causing acute hydronephrosis, common symptoms include severe pain in the back or side(s), swelling in the abdomen, fever, nausea, vomiting, urinary tract infection, need to urinate frequently and painful urination. Chronic hydronephrosis can share the symptoms of the acute disease, but typically it has no symptoms or just an intermittent dull ache in the side. In such cases, chronic kidney failure may be the first sign that the condition exists.

Conventional Medical Treatment: The treatment aims to remove the build up of urine to relieve the pressure on the kidney and treat the cause of the blockage to prevent permanent kidney damage. Catheters can be inserted either into the bladder or the kidney to remove urine, and most blockages require surgery to remove them.

Prognosis: Most make a full recovery. Left untreated it can cause kidney damage or kidney failure.

Holistic Advice: Seek medical attention.

Hyperhidrosis

Definition: Excessive sweating in specific areas (focal hyperhidrosis), typically the feet, armpits, hands and face, or all over the body (generalised hyperhidrosis).

Possible Causes: Can either have no known cause (primary idiopathic hyperhidrosis) or can be symptomatic of an underlying medical condition (secondary hyperhidrosis). Most cases of focal hyperhidrosis are primary idiopathic, whilst the generalised form is usually secondary. It is thought that there is a familial link for primary idiopathic hyperhidrosis and growing evidence to suggest that it may be caused by problems with the sympathetic nervous system. Conditions that can cause secondary hyperhidrosis include hyperthyroidism, pregnancy, anxiety, substance or alcohol abuse, heart disease, respiratory failure, obesity, gout, certain infections, some types of cancer and some neurological conditions. Certain medications, including antidepressants, can also be a trigger.

General Signs and Symptoms: Excessive sweating often accompanied by an unpleasant odour. Primary idiopathic hyperhidrosis usually first appears at puberty.

Conventional Medical Treatment: Secondary (generalised) hyperhidrosis is tackled by treating the underlying condition. There are a variety of treatments for primary (focal) hyperhidrosis including lifestyle changes to improve the symptoms (e.g. avoiding known triggers, wearing antiperspirant and buying clothes made of natural fibres), prescribed antiperspirants containing aluminium chloride (to reduce the activity of the sweat glands), iontophoresis (uses an electric current to block the sweat glands) and injections of botulinum toxin may be advised in some severe cases (but the results are not permanent). If all else fails, minor operations may be performed to destroy the nerve centres that control the sweating.

Prognosis: This condition itself is not considered that serious but it is often accompanied by embarrassment and can cause emotional and psychological distress. The range of treatments is usually effective in controlling the symptoms.

Holistic Advice: Wash regularly and wear loose clothing made from natural fibres. If anxiety is a trigger, relaxation techniques may help.

Hyperparathyroidism

Definition: When the parathyroid produces too much parathyroid hormone causing an increase in blood calcium levels. There are two main types, primary and secondary.

Possible Causes: Primary hyperparathyroidism occurs when there is a problem with the parathyroid gland itself. It is usually caused by a non-cancerous tumour (adenoma) and very rarely by a cancerous tumour. Women are twice as likely to develop primary hyperparathyroidism than men. Secondary hyperparathyroidism occurs when there is nothing wrong with the gland but another condition causes the levels of calcium in the blood to decrease. This is most commonly caused by vitamin D deficiency but can also be cause by kidney failure. Tertiary hyperparathyroidism is rare and associated with very advanced kidney failure.

General Signs and Symptoms: Usually causes few or no symptoms at all. If symptoms are present they are wide ranging and include depression, tiredness, increased thirst, nausea, loss of appetite, muscle weakness, constipation, stomach pain and confusion. When levels of blood calcium are high and left untreated symptoms can include vomiting, dehydration, confusion, muscle spasms, joint/bone pain, heart beat irregularities and hypertension. It is important to note that symptoms are not always directly related to the level of calcium in the blood.

Conventional Medical Treatment: Surgery to remove the parathyroid gland is the most common treatment for primary hyperparathyroidism. If blood calcium levels are very high, bisphosphonates will be prescribed to lower it. This is a short term intervention used prior to surgery. For those unable to have surgery a medication can be prescribed to control the condition. Treatment for secondary hyperparathyroidism is dependent on the cause. Vitamin D supplementation can be used to correct vitamin D deficiency.

Prognosis: Complications are rare but without treatment hyperparathyroidism can lead to osteoporosis, kidney damage, peptic ulcers and pancreatitis. In severe cases kidney failure, coma and serious heart rhythm issues can be developed due to high blood calcium levels.

Holistic Advice: Eat a healthy, balanced diet. Avoid regularly eating foods high in calcium and drink plenty of fluids.

Hypertension

Definition: Persistent high blood pressure (in excess of 140/90mmHg) that may damage the arteries or heart.

Possible Causes: In about 9/10 cases there is no identifiable cause but lifestyle and genetic factors are thought to contribute. Risk factors include age, family history, ethnicity, high fat diet, salt intake, lack of exercise, being overweight, smoking, excessive alcohol consumption and stress. When there is no identifiable cause it is called primary high blood pressure. In other cases the hypertension is caused by an underlying condition. This is called secondary high blood pressure. Underlying conditions that can cause hypertension include kidney conditions, atherosclerosis, some hormonal conditions (e.g. Cushing's syndrome), lupus, some medications (e.g. oral contraceptive pill and nonsteroidal anti-inflammatories) and some recreational drugs.

General Signs and Symptoms: Although usually without symptoms, very high blood pressure can cause headaches, dizziness, blurred vision, tinnitus, shortness of breath and nosebleeds.

Conventional Medical Treatment: Lifestyle changes should be made and, according to the severity of the hypertension and the presence of risk factors, antihypertensive medication may be prescribed. Common blood pressure medications include ACE inhibitors, alpha-blockers, calcium channel blockers, diuretics and beta-blockers.

Prognosis: Hypertension can damage the arteries, heart and kidneys, and is a major risk factor for developing cardiovascular disease. For most, however, medication and lifestyle changes can control the blood pressure and reduce the risk of complications.

Holistic Advice: Reduce intake of saturated fats, salt, tea, coffee and alcohol. Regular exercise, meditation and yoga can be very beneficial. Reduce any excess weight and stop smoking.

Hyperthyroidism

Definition: Overproduction of thyroid hormones. Also called thyrotoxicosis. It is one of the most common hormonal disorders.

Possible Causes: Excess thyroid hormones cause many of the body's functions to speed up. It is commonly caused by Graves' disease. Graves' disease is an autoimmune disorder in which the antibodies attack the thyroid gland, resulting in the overproduction of hormones. It can also be caused by the formation of nodules in the thyroid that increase its hormonal production. Risk factors include family history, excessive iodine in diet, other autoimmune disorders (especially vitiligo (skin condition) and pernicious anaemia, and smoking. Thyroiditis can cause acute attacks.

General Signs and Symptoms: Hyperactivity, sudden weight loss or gain, rapid heartbeat, hand tremors, excessive sweating, intolerance to heat, anxiety, insomnia, frequent bowel movements, swelling in the neck caused by an enlarged thyroid (this is called goitre), and muscle weakness. Those with Graves' disease may also have bulging eyes.

Conventional Medical Treatment: Treatment aims to reduce the amount of thyroid hormones produced. Options include antithyroid drugs, to suppress the production of the thyroid hormones, radioactive iodine, to destroy part of the thyroid, and surgical removal of a part of the thyroid or all of it. Betablockers may be prescribed to counter some of the symptoms such as the hyperactivity, rapid heartbeat and tremors.

Prognosis: Most fully recover. Some treatments may result in the thyroid producing too little thyroid hormones and so hormone supplements may be required. In very rare cases, failure to treat an overactive thyroid may result in a thyroid storm. This is a serious condition that requires urgent medical attention.

Holistic Advice: Thyroid levels should be monitored regularly after treatment. Relaxation techniques may be useful to ease hyperactivity.

Hypoparathyroidism

Definition: A rare conditions where the parathyroid glands produce too little parathyroid hormone causing blood calcium levels to fall.

Possible Causes: The most common cause of hypoparathyroidism is removal of the parathyroid gland or injury to the gland during surgery. Some autoimmune conditions such as Addison's disease and pernicious anaemia can cause the immune system to attack the body's own tissues, causing damage to the parathyroid gland. Some congenital conditions see babies born with without or with low functioning parathyroid glands. Additionally, radiotherapy treatment for throat/neck cancer can damage the parathyroid gland.

General Signs and Symptoms: Symptoms are wide ranging and include tingling in the fingers/toes, muscle twitches in the face, muscle cramps, fatigue, mood swings, dry skin, coarse hair and brittle fingernails.

Conventional Medical Treatment: Treatment aims to relieve symptoms and balance the levels of calcium and other minerals in the blood. Calcium carbonate and vitamin D supplements can be taken to restore calcium levels to normal ranges. In severe cases where blood calcium has dropped significantly, calcium can be administered intravenously. A high-calcium and low phosphorus diet may also be recommended.

Prognosis: Symptoms can be managed with treatment. Taking supplements for hypoparathyroidism is usually for life. Regular blood tests will be required to monitor the levels of calcium, phosphorus and parathyroid hormone levels.

Holistic Advice: Follow a high calcium and low phosphorus diet. High calcium foods include milk, cheese, leafy green vegetables, tofu, soya beans, fortified cereals/bread and nuts. Avoid food containing phosphorus such as red meat, poultry, rice and oats.

Hypotension

Definition: Lower than normal blood pressure.

Possible Causes: Some people naturally have a lower than normal blood pressure and function without any problem. In other cases blood pressure may be reduced for many reasons including the side effect of some medications, heart disease, heart attack, abnormal widening of the blood vessels, serious injury, shock, autonomic disorders (e.g. diabetes mellitus, Parkinson's disease), adrenal problems, infections of the bloodstream (e.g. septicaemia), severe allergic reaction and dehydration. A common form of hypotension is postural hypertension. In this case a fall in blood pressure is experienced when the body's position is changed by suddenly standing or sitting up.

General Signs and Symptoms: Can be asymptomatic unless the pressure is very low. Symptoms may include tiredness, palpitations, weakness, light-headedness, fainting, dizziness, blurred vision and nausea.

Conventional Medical Treatment: Only usually requires treatment if the hypotension is causing symptoms. Treatment depends upon the underlying cause. Medication is rarely prescribed for hypotension.

Prognosis: Low blood pressure, if not problematic, can be of benefit as it can help protect against the conditions associated with hypertension and lessen the risk factors associated with it.

Holistic Advice: Keep hydrated and reduce caffeine and alcohol intake (particularly at night to help avoid dehydration). Eat small, frequent meals. Stand up slowly and wearing support stockings may help.

Hypothyroidism

Definition: A low level of thyroid hormones in the blood.

Possible Causes: In cases of hypothyroidism, the thyroid gland does not produce sufficient quantities of thyroid hormones (particularly thyroxine). This dysfunction of the thyroid is often brought about by an autoimmune reaction that causes the thyroid to become inflamed (thyroiditis), but can also be a side effect of the treatment for hyperthyroidism or of thyroid cancer. Severe iodine deficiency, the reaction of the thyroid to viruses or drugs, abnormal thyroid development and a problem with the pituitary gland may also rarely cause this condition.

General Signs and Symptoms: A low level of thyroxine slows many body functions. This causes weight gain, muscle aches and extreme tiredness. Other early symptoms include cramps, sensitivity to cold, constipation, slowness in body and mind, muscle weakness, dry skin, brittle hair and nails, heavy or irregular periods and depression. It may be present from birth but is more common in the over 40's, particularly women. Symptoms have a gradual onset. In very rare cases, severe hypothyroidism can lead to myxoedema coma, a life threatening condition. This causes confusion, hypothermia and drowsiness.

Conventional Medical Treatment: Thyroxine tablets are used to rebalance the deficiency. The amount given should be regularly monitored. Myxoedema coma requires emergency hospital treatment and replacement of the thyroid hormone intravenously. In some cases of myxoedema coma breathing support, steroid mediation and antibiotics will also be required.

Prognosis: It is a lifelong disorder but taking thyroxine will cure the symptoms. Untreated hypothyroidism can lead to myxoedema coma, which is life threatening.

Holistic Advice: Exercise regularly and maintain a balanced diet. Include white fish, shellfish, dairy and sea vegetables (e.g. seaweed) as a source of iodine if required.

Hysterectomy

Definition: Surgical procedure to remove the uterus.

Possible Causes: Hysterectomies are conducted to treat a number of health problems. It is often only considered when less invasive treatments have been tried without success.

General Signs and Symptoms: Women considering a hysterectomy may have heavy periods, chronic pelvic pain from endometriosis or pelvic inflammatory disease, fibroids (non-cancerous tumours), uterine prolapse, ovarian cancer, uterine cancer, cervical cancer and cancer of the fallopian tubes.

Conventional Medical Treatment: There are many types of hysterectomy and the procedure that is carried out will depend on why the operation is being performed and how much of the surrounding organs can be safely left in place. The main types are; total hysterectomy (womb and cervix are removed), subtotal hysterectomy (main body of the womb is removed, cervix left in place), total hysterectomy with bilateral salpingo-oophorectomy (womb, cervix, fallopian tubes and ovaries are removed) and radical hysterectomy (womb and surround tissues removed including fallopian tubes, part of the vagina, ovaries, lymph glands and fatty tissue).

Prognosis: A major operation with a long recovery time of approximately 6 – 8 weeks. Complications can include bleeding, damage to the bladder, bowel or ureter, infection, blood clots and ovary failure. If the ovaries are removed then surgical menopause will occur.

Holistic Advice: After surgery, rest as much as possible to allow the musculature and surround tissues to heal properly. Avoid heavy lifting.

Impetigo

Definition: A common and highly contagious skin infection.

Possible Causes: Bacterial infection of the skin caused by the Staphylococcus aureus or Streptococcus pyogenes bacteria. The bacteria can enter otherwise healthy skin via a cut, insect bite or injury (primary impetigo). Underlying conditions that cause damage to the skin such as head lice, scabies or eczema can also allow bacteria to enter (secondary impetigo). Most common in children and those with a low resistance to infection such as diabetics or those with HIV. The condition spread very easily by direct physical contact and by sharing towels or bedding.

General Signs and Symptoms: Non-bullous impetigo is characterised by red sores, most commonly around the nose and mouth. The sores can be itchy or painful and quickly burst leaving thick golden crusts, much like cornflakes, on the skin. As the crusts dry and fall off they leave a red mark that fades over time. Bullous impetigo is characterised by 1-2cm wide fluid filled blisters on the trunk of the body or arms and legs. Spreading quickly the blisters will eventually burst, leaving a yellow crust. The blister can be painful and itchy. In both types of impetigo there can be symptoms of fever and swollen glands but it is more common in bullous.

Conventional Medical Treatment: Can resolve on its own however, treatment is highly recommended as it promotes healing and limits the risk of the infection being spread to others. Topical antibiotics are most common though oral antibiotics may be prescribed in more severe cases. If recurring, an antiseptic nasal cream may be prescribed.

Prognosis: Symptoms usually clear up after 2 – 3 weeks without treatment and between 7 – 10 days with treatment. Scarring can occur if the sores/blisters/crusts are picked or scratched. Complications are rare and can include cellulitis, scarlet fever and sepsis.

Holistic Advice: Keep any breaks in the skin clean. Wash your hands regularly and wash any clothes, bedding or towels that have had contact with the affected areas. Keep affected areas dry and covered with loose clothing or a bandage.

Impotence

Definition: Inability to achieve or sustain an erection. Called erectile dysfunction.

Possible Causes: Occasional impotence is normal, but persistent, long-term difficulty in achieving an erection may indicate an underlying problem. It can be caused by either a physical or psychological cause, or a combination of the two. Men who are impotent with their partners, but are able to achieve erection by masturbation or wake up with an erection, are likely to have a psychological reason for the condition, e.g. anxiety, depression, relationship difficulties or the fear of failure. If an erection is not achievable under any circumstances, the cause is more likely to be physical. Conditions that may cause impotence can be those that affect blood flow to the penis (e.g. cardiovascular disease, hypertension, high cholesterol, diabetes), those that affect the nervous system (e.g. multiple sclerosis, Parkinson's disease) and hormonal conditions such as hypogonadism (which causes low levels of testosterone), hyperthyroidism and hypothyroidism. Some anatomical conditions can also affect the penile tissue. Impotence may also be a side effect of some drugs, including certain antidepressants, diuretics and antihypertensives. Risk factors include tiredness, heavy drinking, smoking and the use of illegal drugs.

General Signs and Symptoms: The inability to get and sustain an erection sufficient for satisfactory sexual intercourse.

Conventional Medical Treatment: Treatment will depend upon the underlying cause. If impotence is due to a physical condition, successfully treating that condition is likely to help. In cases caused by psychological problems, there are various forms of psychological treatments such as psychosexual counselling that may be of benefit. A variety of drugs are available to temporarily increase the blood flow to the penis (e.g. Viagra). Blood can also be encouraged to the penis with the use of a vacuum pump. Lifestyle changes to reduce the risk factors are important and they often help reduce the symptoms. Penile implants are usually only considered for those whose impotence is caused by pelvic trauma or anatomical penile problems.

Prognosis: In many cases it can be successfully treated. It can impact on the quality of life of the sufferer and his partner.

Holistic Advice: Although it is seen as an embarrassing condition, men should be encouraged to seek medical advice rather than trying to deal with it themselves.

Indigestion

Definition: Pain or discomfort in the upper abdomen, usually after eating. Also known as dyspepsia.

Possible Causes: Stomach acid comes into contact with the sensitive lining of the digestive tract, causing irritation and inflammation. It is usually associated with eating but can also be caused by infection and the reaction to certain medications. Indigestion can also be symptomatic of another condition such as gastro-oesophageal reflux, peptic ulcers or, in rare cases, stomach cancer.

General Signs and Symptoms: Symptoms include feeling bloated, heartburn, nausea and belching. Risk factors include smoking and being overweight. May be triggered by certain foods, e.g. rich, fatty, heavily spiced food, overeating, drinking excess coffee or alcohol, eating too quickly and stress.

Conventional Medical Treatment: Changes to diet and lifestyle can often reduce attacks, and antacids are usually sufficient to relieve the symptoms. A variety of other drugs to counter stomach acidity are available. If symptoms persist, worsen or are accompanied by vomiting, loss of appetite or loss of weight, a Doctor should be consulted as these can be signs of a more serious condition. Once identified, the underlying condition can then be treated, hopefully reducing the indigestion.

Prognosis: Changes to diet and lifestyle are usually sufficient unless there is an underlying medical condition. Persistent irritation of the digestive tract by stomach acid can cause serious problems.

Holistic Advice: Eat smaller portions at regular intervals, and do not eat within 3 hours of bedtime. Reduce caffeine and alcohol intake. Keep a food diary to try to ascertain any dietary triggers. Lose any excess weight and do not smoke. If possible (and, if necessary, agreed by a Doctor) avoid medicines that are known to irritate the digestive tract (e.g. aspirin).

Inflamed Gallbladder

Definition: Inflammation of the gallbladder. Also known by the medical term acute cholecystitis. Can be grouped into two categories calculous cholecystitis and acalculous cholecystitis.

Possible Causes: Usually caused by a gallstone blocking the cystic duct. Calculous cholecystitis is most common, usually less serious and occurs when the cystic duct is blocked by a gallstone or biliary sludge. Acalculous cholecystitis is less common, usually more serious and is often a complication of serious illness, infection or injury to the gallbladder. Being overweight, particularly obese, increases the risk of gallstones and therefore increases the chance of a blockage forming.

General Signs and Symptoms: The main symptom is a sharp, sudden pain in the upper right hand side of the abdomen which can spread to toward the right shoulder. Pain will persist and the area will be tender to the touch. Additional symptoms include fever, nausea, vomiting, sweating, jaundice, sweating and a visible bulge in the abdomen.

Conventional Medical Treatment: Hospitalisation is often required. Initial treatment may include fasting, intravenous fluids and painkillers. If infection is suspected then antibiotics will be prescribed. After initial treatment it may be recommended to surgically remove the gallbladder (cholecystectomy) to eliminate the risk of the condition reoccurring.

Prognosis: Without treatment there can be life-threatening complications such as gangrenous cholecystitis, where the tissue of the gallbladder dies increasing the risk of serious infection. The gallbladder may also split (perforated gallbladder) potentially spreading infection within the abdominal cavity (peritonitis) or cause an abscess. Removal of the gallbladder via surgery still allows the person to lead a normal life.

Holistic Advice: Adopt and maintain a healthy, balanced diet and reduce high-cholesterol foods. Maintain a healthy weight and take regular exercise. Gradual weight loss plans are recommended for those who need to lose weight.

Influenza

Definition: Infection of the upper respiratory tract. Commonly called seasonal flu.

Possible Causes: Caused by the influenza virus. The infection is highly contagious and is spread both in airborne droplets from coughs and sneezes and by direct contact. The flu virus can mutate, producing new strains to which few will have immunity.

General Signs and Symptoms: Symptoms develop 24-48 hours after infection. Symptoms usually include fever, sweating, shivering, aching muscles, exhaustion, sneezing, runny or stuffy nose, sore throat, cough and loss of appetite.

Conventional Medical Treatment: Bed rest, plenty of fluids and painkillers such as paracetamol can relieve the symptoms in most cases. Over-the-counter cold and flu remedies are also available. Medical attention should be sought if breathing problems arise, if the fever lasts for more than a couple of days or if a rash develops.

Prognosis: Symptoms usually clear up in about 5-8 days. Can be dangerous to the elderly.

Holistic Advice: The elderly and vulnerable groups can be immunized. Ensure good hand hygiene to help avoid contracting or spreading the virus. Honey and lemon drinks can be soothing. Eat a healthy, balanced diet. Boost the immune system.

Ingrown Hair

Definition: A condition where a hair has grown back into the skin.

Possible Causes: Most commonly due to shaving though waxing, plucking and threading can all cause ingrown hairs. The face, neck, legs, armpits and pubic area are most susceptible. Coarse or curly hair is more likely to become ingrown.

General Signs and Symptoms: Usually present as red, raised, itchy spots on the skin. The hair maybe visibly trapped. If infected, pus will be present and it may cause pain/discomfort.

Conventional Medical Treatment: Usually require little to no treatment. Creams and lotions can be used to prevent itching. Exfoliating scrubs can be used to free trapped hairs. Mild antiseptic creams can be used to help present infection. If the ingrown hair is particularly bad a Doctor or Nurse may use a needle or scalpel to free the hair. Steroid creams to help with swelling and antibiotic creams/tablets to treat infection may also be prescribed.

Prognosis: Usually resolve by themselves. Chronic ingrown hairs can lead to infection or scarring.

Holistic Advice: Prevention is key. Always use a sharp razor, or, alternatively look for longer-term methods of hair removal such as laser or electrolysis.

Ingrown Nail

Definition: A condition in which the edge of a nail grows into the skin. Also known as onychocryptosis.

Possible Causes: Cutting nails too short, cutting the edges of the nails, tight fitting footwear, and injury to the digit can cause this condition. If the skin is warm and moist there is more chance of ingrown nails, so excessive sweating of the feet or poor hygiene may increase the incidence. Genetic factors that influence posture, gait, or the shape of the digits and nails may also contribute.

General Signs and Symptoms: Area where the nail has pierced the skin becomes red, swollen, inflamed and may bleed. The big toe is the most likely to suffer. If left untreated the digits can become infected.

Conventional Medical Treatment: In mild cases treated early, foot baths may enable the skin to be pushed back. Alternatively the part of the nail that is growing into the digit, or the whole nail, may need to be surgically removed. Painkillers may be required for the pain and antibiotics to clear any infection.

Prognosis: Very painful at the time but no lasting significant consequences.

Holistic Advice: Cut nails in a straight line, not with rounded edges. Wear shoes and socks that fit. See a GP or podiatrist as soon as a problem becomes evident.

Insomnia

Definition: Regular inability to fall asleep or stay asleep.

Possible Causes: Can be caused simply by trying to sleep in a noisy environment, but it is commonly triggered by factors such as worry, anxiety, a high intake of caffeine, alcohol and nicotine, and drug abuse. Regular sleep patterns can become quickly lost, and the insomnia becomes habitual. Insomnia can be symptomatic of some conditions that cause problems of a night such as asthma, hyperthyroidism, heart disease, incontinence and arthritis, and pain may also cause the person to wake up prematurely. Insomnia is also often associated with mental health problems such as depression, mood disorders, psychotic disorders, and anxiety disorders. Some medications can cause insomnia, e.g. antidepressants, drugs for hypertension, antiepileptic drugs and non-steroidal anti-inflammatories. Insomnia is more common in women and in the elderly.

General Signs and Symptoms: Inability to go to sleep or waking during the night and being unable to get back to sleep. It can be a distressing and frustrating condition, leading to excessive tiredness, irritability and a general inability to cope. It can lead to a greater risk of accidents.

Conventional Medical Treatment: The triggers need to be tackled. Changes in lifestyle, such as taking more exercise and drinking less alcohol and caffeine, can be of benefit. Guidance will be given on how to promote good sleeping patterns, such as keeping regular bedtimes, avoiding food late at night and trying to relax before bedtime. Sleeping tablets can be used short-term to help restore the sleeping pattern but should not be taken long-term. Cognitive and behavioural treatments may be of use to change thoughts and behaviour patterns that may be worsening the problem.

Prognosis: If caused by an underlying medical condition, then treating that will often help. Tackling any worries or anxieties, making life style changes and creating a bedtime routine will usually help the insomnia to disappear.

Holistic Advice: Ensure the bedroom is a relaxing, calm environment that is conducive to sleep. Avoid watching television or using electric equipment such as mobile phones and computers just before bedtime, and try not to have them in the bedroom. Develop a bedtime routine. Take regular exercise, eat a balanced, healthy diet and avoid alcohol, caffeine and spicy foods (particularly just before bedtime). Give up smoking.

Irritable Bowel Syndrome

Definition: Chronic condition of the digestive system causing intermittent abdominal pain, diarrhoea and constipation. Abbreviated to IBS.

Possible Causes: The exact cause of IBS is not know but possible physical and psychological contributing factors include the abnormal contraction of the muscles in the intestinal walls, sensitivity of the digestive organs to pain, immune system problems, problems with how the central nervous system controls the digestive system, an unusual response to infection, sensitivity to certain foods, environmental and genetic factors, stress and depression.

General Signs and Symptoms: Common symptoms can include abdominal pain, changes in bowel habits, bloating and swelling of the abdomen, a feeling of fullness and difficulty in finishing meals, excessive wind, nausea and vomiting, an urgent need to defaecate, feeling that the bowel has not fully emptied after defaecation and the passing of mucus from the rectum. Symptoms are usually worse after eating and can fluctuate in severity, with periods of remission and relapse. Other symptoms may include lower back pain, muscle and joint pain, constant tiredness, headache, belching, halitosis and a frequent and urgent need to urinate. IBS is twice as common in women then men and normally develops between the ages of 20-30 but can affect any age.

Conventional Medical Treatment: There is no cure but the symptoms can often be controlled by a combination of lifestyle and dietary changes and relaxation techniques. If symptoms persist medication may be required to treat the symptoms. Antispasmodic medicines (to reduce abdominal pain and cramping), laxatives (to combat constipation), antimotility medicines (to treat diarrhoea) and tricyclic antidepressants (to reduce abdominal pain and cramping) may be prescribed. Psychological therapies may also be used to help control the condition.

Prognosis: IBS poses no serious threat to health, but there is a need to rule out other more serious digestive disorders which display similar symptoms.

Holistic Advice: Keep a food diary to try to identify any dietary triggers. Eat regularly, drink plenty of water and reduce alcohol and coffee consumption. Probiotics may help. Exercise regularly to keep fit and defuse stress. Anything that reduces stress, such as relaxation techniques and yoga, may help. Acupuncture, reflexology and aloe vera (a herbal remedy) may be of benefit.

Jaundice

Definition: Yellow discoloration of the skin and the whites of the eyes. It is a symptom of disease, not a condition itself.

Possible Causes: Jaundice results from excessively high levels of a yellowish pigment called bilirubin in the blood. Bilirubin originates in the red blood cells. The liver breaks down bilirubin and excretes it. If for any reason the liver cannot remove the bilirubin, jaundice occurs. There are 3 main reasons for jaundice - 1. In hepatocellular jaundice, the liver is damaged and unable to process the bilirubin. 2. In haemolytic jaundice, too many red blood cells are broken down so the liver can't cope with the quantity of bilirubin in the blood. 3. In obstructive jaundice, the bile duct is blocked, causing a backlog of bilirubin in the liver which is forced back into the blood. Jaundice can be a symptom of many disorders of the liver, gall bladder, and pancreas. It may also be caused by some blood disorders. Jaundice is common in a newly born baby if the liver is not fully functional. This usually resolves in about a week.

General Signs and Symptoms: Yellow discoloration of the skin and the whites of the eyes. The body fluids may also appear discolored. Depending on the cause of the jaundice, symptoms may also include tiredness, abdominal pain, itchy skin, vomiting, weight loss and fever.

Conventional Medical Treatment: Investigation is always required to establish the underlying medical condition that is causing the jaundice. If the underlying condition can be treated, the jaundice will disappear.

Prognosis: Depends upon the underlying condition.

Holistic Advice: Take measures to keep the liver healthy, such as drinking plenty of fluids, reducing alcohol intake, maintaining a healthy, balanced diet, and taking regular exercise.

Kidney Stones

Definition: Crystallized deposits that build up in the one or both of the kidneys. Also called nephrolithiasis.

Possible Causes: Crystallization of waste products in the kidney which, over time, build up into a hard stone. They are usually formed following a build up of calcium (the most common type), ammonia, uric acid or cystine. The exact cause is unknown but risk factors include insufficient fluid intake, immobility, family history, repeated urinary infections, history of kidney stones, only having one kidney and diseases of the small intestine. Medications such as aspirin, antacids, and calcium and vitamin D supplements can also increase the risk, as does the treatment used for certain medical conditions such as cancer or kidney disease.

General Signs and Symptoms: Small stones often pass unnoticed. Symptoms only tend to be caused if the stone gets stuck in the kidney, when it travels down the ureter, or if it causes an infection. Symptoms of kidney stones are collectively referred to as renal colic and include severe pain in the back or side of the abdomen, restlessness, nausea, vomiting, blood in the urine, cloudy or smelly urine, burning sensation on urination, fever and a feeling that urination is necessary even if it is not. If the stone is passed in the urine the pain rapidly subsides. However, if they get stuck hydronephrosis and kidney infections can be caused.

Conventional Medical Treatment: The treatment depends on the stone. Small stones may just pass in the urine and medication can be taken to relieve the pain, nausea and vomiting. Large stones may need treatment to remove them. The most common treatment is lithotripsy, which involves sending high-energy shock waves through the stone to break it up. Percutaneous nephrolithotomy is a technique in which a nephroscope is passed into the kidney to remove the stone. Ureterorenoscopy techniques can be used to remove a stone from a ureter. For large stones conventional surgery is sometimes required.

Prognosis: Complications are rare but kidney stones often recur.

Holistic Advice: Those prone to stones should drink up 2-3 litres of fluid a day, especially during hot weather or when perspiring. Dehydration will increase the concentration of the urine, so increasing the risk of kidney stones and disorders such as cystitis. Empty the bladder as soon as you need to because the longer the urine remains in the body, the more likely it is that the minerals will crystallize. Dietary changes may help according to the type of stone.

Laryngitis

Definition: Inflammation of the larynx.

Possible Causes: Acute laryngitis is usually caused by a viral Infection (e.g. the common cold or flu) or physical injury (caused by shouting, prolonged singing or by swallowing very hot fluids). Chronic laryngitis can be caused by smoking, alcohol misuse, gastro-oesophageal reflux, and a range of environmental factors (e.g. long term exposure to dust, fumes and chemicals). Dry air from central heating can aggravate the condition.

General Signs and Symptoms: The larynx appears red and swollen. This is accompanied by hoarseness or a complete loss of the voice, sore painful throat, mild fever, a loud, barking, rough or husky cough, and a constant need to clear the throat. Inspiration and expiration can be difficult, particularly in children.

Conventional Medical Treatment: Acute laryngitis has no medical treatment as such. Resting the vocal cords, keeping hydrated and boosting the immune system are recommended. Antibiotics will only be given if there is a bacterial infection. Chronic laryngitis is treated according to its cause. Mostly this will involve lifestyle changes.

Prognosis: Most sufferers of acute laryngitis will make a full recovery without any complications. Chronic laryngitis takes longer to clear and can cause permanent damage.

Holistic Advice: Rest the voice. If laryngitis is due to an infection following a cold, cough or sore throat, then look at boosting the immune system. Steam inhalation may be of benefit. Stop smoking, avoid smoky environments and reduce alcohol intake. Laryngitis can cause great frustration as well as discomfort, so treat the whole person.

Leg Ulcer

Definition: A persistent open sore, usually on the lower part of the leg.

Possible Causes: Leg ulcers commonly occur when the skin breaks down due to poor circulation. An open sore then develops, either spontaneously or following a minor injury. There are several types of leg ulcer: venous (sometimes referred to as stasis or varicose) – occur on the veins, arterial – occur on the arteries, diabetic – occur due to high blood sugar associated with diabetes, vasculitic – due to chronic inflammatory disorders, traumatic – caused by injury, and malignant – caused by a skin tumour. Venous leg ulcers are the most common. Risk factors include compromised circulation, age, immobility, diabetes, obesity, deep vein thrombosis and varicose veins.

General Signs and Symptoms: Initially there is pain, itching and swelling on the affected leg. The skin breaks and the ulcer appears as a shallow, pink area of broken skin. The surrounding tissue may be swollen. They are often painful and very slow to heal.

Conventional Medical Treatment: The ulcers are cleaned and dressed. Compression bandages may be used to help control the blood pressure in the legs. The underlying reason for the ulcer will be addressed. If the ulcer becomes infected, antibiotics may be prescribed.

Prognosis: May take several months to heal. If circulation or immobility is not improved they may return.

Holistic Advice: Take regular exercise to improve circulation. Lose any excess weight and stop smoking. Keep the legs moisturised and inspect them regularly for signs of skin damage.

Leukaemia

Definition: Cancer of the white blood cells. There are many different types, for example, acute myeloid leukaemia, acute lymphoblastic leukaemia, chronic myeloid leukaemia and chronic lymphocytic leukaemia. Note: Acute or chronic does not describe how serious the disease is, but how quickly it will progress.

Possible Causes: An overproduction of abnormal white blood cells, specifically myeloid or lymphoid stem cells. Due to build-up of abnormal cells in the bone marrow, the production of normal cells is disrupted. In the majority of cases, there is no clear cause. Risk factors include older age, being male and bone marrow disorders. Less commonly previous family history of leukaemia or exposure to high levels of radiation/chemicals can increase risk of developing leukaemia.

General Signs and Symptoms: Symptoms are often vague. A lack of red blood cells can cause weakness, tiredness, shortness of breath and palpitations. Regular and more severe infections can occur due to lack of healthy white blood cells. A reduction in platelets can cause bleeding and bruising. Some leukaemia's can cause swollen glands.

Conventional Medical Treatment: The main treatments are chemotherapy and radiotherapy. Sometimes targeted therapy and biological therapy is used. Acute leukaemia will usually require immediate intensive treatment. Some younger or very fit people with acute leukaemia can be offered a stem cell transplant as an alternative to chemotherapy. In some chronic leukaemia's, 'active surveillance' will be used first as the cancer develops slowly.

Prognosis: Overall, treatment for acute leukaemia is very effective and most will go into remission. Chronic leukaemia is not often 'curable' but treatable. Chronic leukaemia may return more readily. Some people will experience long term problems including a weakened immune system, bleeding (due to low platelet levels) and infertility.

Holistic Advice: Take steps to boost the immune system. Avoid infection by practicing good food and hand hygiene.

Liver Cancer

Definition: Cancer found anywhere in the liver. Hepatocellular carcinoma (HCC) is the most common and covered below.

Possible Causes: Causes of liver cancer are not always clear but there are risk factors that increase the chance of developing it. It is more common in men and people over the age of 60. Previous damage to the liver caused by cirrhosis or conditions such as HIV, gallstones, hepatitis B or C and diabetes all increase the chance of cancer developing. Lifestyle factors such as being overweight or obese, smoking, heavy alcohol use and exposure to certain chemicals increase risk of disease. Family history of the disease is also a risk factor.

General Signs and Symptoms: Liver cancer does not always cause symptoms and when they occur they can be non-specific. Symptoms can include weight loss, jaundice, itching, nausea, indigestion, pain and swelling in the abdomen and a loss of appetite. Generally feeing unwell or persistent tiredness may also be experienced. The symptoms are the same if the cancer started in the liver (primary) or spread from another area (secondary).

Conventional Medical Treatment: Dependent on the size, type and location of the cancer as well as if the cancer is primary or secondary. If the cancer is primary and still small surgery is recommended to remove part or all of the liver. Chemotherapy and radiotherapy can be used to kill cancer cells and stop them coming back. Thermal ablation, the use of heat to destroy cancer cells, may be recommended if surgery is not an option. Targeted cancer medication can also be used to slow the growth of the cancer surgery is not an option or the cancer has spread.

Prognosis: Dependent on the size, type and location of the cancer as well as if the cancer is primary or secondary.

Holistic Advice: Stop smoking and lose weight if required. Reduce alcohol consumption and eat a healthy balanced diet.

Lung Cancer

Definition: Cancer of the lungs. Two main types are classified by the cells where the cancer starts growing; non-small-cell lung cancer (most common) and small-cell lung cancer (less common and spreads faster).

Possible Causes: The most common cause of lung cancer is smoking cigarettes. Tobacco contains toxic substances that are known to be carcinogenic. Therefore, smoking cigars, pipes and using snuff, chewing tobacco and even passive smoking can also increase the risk of developing lung cancer. Exposure to chemicals and substances such as radon, arsenic, asbestos, coal and silica can cause damage to the lungs and increase the risk of cancer. Lung cancer is more common in older adults ages 75 and over.

General Signs and Symptoms: Early stages of lung cancer often have no signs or symptoms. The main symptoms develop as the cancer progresses and includes a persistent cough, reoccurring chest infections, coughing up blood, pain when breathing or coughing and persistent breathlessness. Fatigue and unexplained weight loss are also common. Less common symptoms are clubbing of the fingers, swelling of the face/neck, difficulty swallowing, wheezing and persistent chest/shoulder pain.

Conventional Medical Treatment: Dependent on the type, size and stage of the cancer. The overall health of the person will also be taken into account. If in good health, with non-small-cell lung cancer in one lung, surgery can be used to remove the cancer followed by chemotherapy. The three types of surgery available for lung cancer; lobectomy, pneumonectomy and wedge resection or segmentectomy. If the non-small-cell cancer has spread a little, with surgery not possible, a course of radiotherapy may be offered. A large spread of non-small-cell cancer will require chemotherapy and/or immunotherapy. Small-cell cancer is most commonly treated with chemotherapy, sometimes in combination with radiotherapy. In rare cases surgery can be used for small-cell cancer, however, the cancer has usually already spread making it an inappropriate treatment.

Prognosis: Dependent on the type, stage and treatment received. As with many cancers, if caught and treated early there is a good chance of remission.

Holistic Advice: Stop smoking. Eat a healthy balanced diet and exercise regularly.

Lupus

Definition: Chronic autoimmune condition that causes inflammation in the body's tissues. There are 2 main types. The most common is systemic lupus erythematosus (SLE) which affects the whole body. Discoid lupus erythematosus only affects the skin. SLE is covered below.

Possible Causes: In this autoimmune condition the body produces antibodies that react against its own connective tissues causing them to become inflamed and swollen. The exact cause is unknown but it is thought to be a combination of genetic and environmental factors. Possible triggers include viruses, infections, some medications, exposure to sunlight, hormonal changes and childbirth.

General Signs and Symptoms: The condition is characterized by intermittent flare ups of joint pain (particularly in the hands and feet), fatigue and skin rashes (commonly on the face, wrists and hands). Other possible symptoms include fever, changes in weight, swollen glands, recurring mouth ulcers, alopecia, hypertension, migraine, anaemia, Raynaud's disease (which limits the blood supply to the hands), increased sensitivity to sunlight, depression and anxiety. Symptoms vary from person to person and range from mild to severe.

Conventional Medical Treatment: Lupus may be treated with non-steroidal anti-inflammatories, hydroxychloroquine, cortiosteroids and immunosuppressants.

Prognosis: There is no cure but the treatments can usually manage the symptoms. For some sufferers, lupus can lead to more serious conditions such as kidney damage, other autoimmune conditions, blood and heart conditions, and pleurisy.

Holistic Advice: Protect the skin and eyes from the sun. Physiotherapy may be useful for joint problems.

Lymphadenopathy/Lymphadenitis

Definition: Enlarged lymph nodes.

Possible Causes: Lymph nodes most commonly become swollen due to a bacterial or viral infection (lymphadenitis). The lymph nodes in the neck, groin and armpits are closer to the surface and so these are the ones that are usually noticed. The swelling will usually subside when the infection clears up. Many conditions caused by infection will have lymphadenopathy as a symptom, for example the lymph nodes in the neck commonly swell during tonsillitis. Some medical conditions can cause long term lymphadenopathy, e.g. tuberculosis and AIDS. Persistent swelling of many or all the lymph nodes may be indicative some types of cancer such as breast cancer, lymphoma and leukaemia.

General Signs and Symptoms: Swollen and sometime painful lymph nodes. When caused by cancer, the swollen lymph nodes do not usually feel painful.

Conventional Medical Treatment: Treating the underlying cause will usually cure this condition. Antibiotics can help bacterial infections.

Prognosis: No complications unless caused by a serious underlying condition.

Holistic Advice: Boost the immune system to help the body combat the infection.

Lymphoedema

Definition: Localised accumulation of fluid in the lymphatic vessels causing swelling in the body's tissues.

Possible Causes: Lymphoedema is caused by damage or disruption to the lymphatic system which renders it unable to successfully drain fluid away from the tissues. The excess fluid accumulates in the tissues and causes the tissues to swell. There are 2 types - primary, which is caused by faulty genes and develops at birth or shortly after puberty and, more commonly, secondary, which may be caused by infection (especially cellulitis), inflammatory diseases (e.g. rheumatoid arthritis, dermatitis and eczema), cardiovascular diseases (e.g. deep vein thrombosis and venous leg ulcers), cancer of the lymphatic system, cancer treatments that cause harm the lymphatic system, trauma and injury.

General Signs and Symptoms: Typically the swelling is in the arms or legs but other places may be affected. Limbs may feel heavy, lose mobility and be painful. There may be tingling, skin infections and skin conditions such as blisters and wart-like growths.

Conventional Medical Treatment: Manual lymphatic drainage, multilayer lymphoedema bandaging, remedial exercises and skin care combine to help treat the symptoms. Surgery may be possible in the form of liposuction to remove excess fat from the area which can reduce the swelling.

Prognosis: Lymphoedema is a life long disorder with no cure, but symptoms can usually be controlled using a combination of treatments. Any damage to the skin can quickly lead to infection and be slow to heal. Sufferers run a high risk of cellulitis which can be treated with antibiotics.

Holistic Advice: Take great care with the skin, lose excess weight and maintain a healthy diet. Avoid alcohol and spicy food as they may increase swelling. Air travel may also worsen the condition. Elevate the affected limbs when possible. Sufferers are often very aware that the conditions has a negative effect on appearance and so they may be self-conscious, stressed and depressed.

Lymphoma

Definition: Cancer that develops in the lymphatic system.

Possible Causes: A mutation in a subset of the white blood cells, which causes them to multiply uncontrollably. There are two main types, non-Hodgkin lymphoma and Hodgkin lymphoma. The exact cause of lymphoma is unknown.

General Signs and Symptoms: The most common symptom are painless swellings in the neck, armpit or groin. This is caused by excess lymphocytes collecting in the lymph nodes. Sometimes there will be more generalised symptoms such as night sweats, fatigue, unexpected weight loss, fever and an itching sensation over the skin.

Conventional Medical Treatment: Treatment will depend on the type, stage and location of the cancer. General health will also be taken into consideration.

Prognosis: Dependent on the type of lymphoma. Some people will experience long-term problems including a weakened immune system, infertility and secondary cancers. The risk of developing cardiovascular and lung disease increases after having lymphoma.

Holistic Advice: Maintain a healthy weight and keep active. Take steps to boost the immune system.

Mastitis

Definition: Inflammation of the breast tissue.

Possible Causes: The most common cause is milk not being completely removed from the breast during breastfeeding. It commonly occurs in the first 6 weeks of breastfeeding but it can also develop if breastfeeding is suddenly stopped and the breasts become overfilled with milk. There are 2 main types - non-infectious, which is caused by the surplus milk blocking the milk ducts, and infectious, which is caused by a bacterial infection. Left untreated non-infectious mastitis can become infectious, due to bacteria infecting the remaining milk. Mastitis can also be experienced by non-breastfeeding women and is caused by bacterial infection. It is more common in smokers and those pre and post menopause.

General Signs and Symptoms: Breast tissue becomes swollen, sore, red, hard, and may feel lumpy. It usually only affects one area of a breast. There may be flu-like symptoms with a fever and chills. There may be a discharge from the nipple.

Conventional Medical Treatment: The continuation of breast feeding will help to remove the blocked milk and improve the symptoms. Advice may be given on breastfeeding techniques. Painkillers can be taken to ease the pain and warm compresses on the affected part of the breast may give relief. Infectious mastitis may need antibiotics.

Prognosis: Left untreated the inflammation caused by infectious mastitis can worsen and a breast abscess may develop.

Holistic Advice: Take rest and drink plenty of fluids. Any breast lumps or noticeable changes in the breast tissue should be examined by a Doctor.

Melasma

Definition: A common skin condition in adults causing patches of pigmentation. Also known as cholasma or pregnancy mask.

Possible Causes: Exact cause is unknown. It is thought to be caused by melanocytes (pigment producing cells) producing too much melanin (pigment). Factors that are thought to increase the chance of melisma developing include pregnancy, use of contraceptive pill, hormone replacement therapy, sun exposure and family history of the condition. Melasma is more common in women, people of colour and people who tan easily.

General Signs and Symptoms: Melasma mainly affects the face but can also appear on areas of the body regularly exposed to the sun, like the forearms or neck. The affected areas will become darker than the surrounding skin. This condition has no physical symptoms but can be psychologically or emotionally distressing.

Conventional Medical Treatment: Treatment aims to improve the appearance of the affected areas. High factor sun creams can reduce the chance of melasma darkening further during sun exposure. Retinoid and hydroquinone creams can help the appearance of the darkened areas. Skin camouflage crème can be used to hide the darker areas. More invasive procedures such as chemical peel, microneedling and laser therapy may also be recommend.

Prognosis: There is currently no cure for melasma but treatment can help to improve the appearance of the condition. Melasma often recurs when treatment is stopped. If melasma occurs during pregnancy it may disappear once the baby has been born.

Holistic Advice: Avoid known triggers such as the contraceptive pill, hormone replacement therapy, tanning beds and sun exposure. Use high SPF sun creams.

Meningitis

Definition: Inflammation of the meninges (the membranes that cover the brain and spinal cord).

Possible Causes: Most often caused by a bacterial or viral infection of the meninges. The infection causes the meninges to swell, which can lead to nerve and brain damage. Bacterial meningitis is the most serious and should be treated as a medical emergency. It is most commonly caused by the meningococcal bacteria or the streptococcus bacteria. If left untreated it can lead to serious brain damage and blood poisoning. It is spread by coughing, sneezing, sharing objects that have been in the mouth, such as cutlery, toothbrushes and cigarettes. Viral meningitis is the most common type and is often mistaken for flu. The virus (commonly enteroviruses or herpes simplex) is spread by coughing, sneezing and contact with contaminated objects. Those with a weakened immune system are at greater risk of contracting all types of meningitis.

General Signs and Symptoms: The symptoms of bacterial meningitis have a rapid onset and quickly worsen. In adults, meningitis may first show as mild fever with general aches and pains, and the skin may appear pale or blotchy. The symptoms then rapidly progress and may include severe headache, vomiting, fever, stiff neck, sensitivity to light, drowsiness, confusion and fits. There may be a distinctive reddish-purple skin rash that does not disappear when pressed. Babies may appear unresponsive and floppy or stiff and jerky, be very sleepy, adopt a staring expression, have a loss of appetite, vomit, have pale and blotchy skin, cry and be irritable but not want to be held. Most with viral meningitis show only flu-like symptoms but in severe cases a stiff neck, muscle and joint pain, nausea, vomiting, diarrhoea, and sensitivity to light may be experienced.

Conventional Medical Treatment: Intravenous antibiotics are used to treat bacterial meningitis. The patient will need to be monitored carefully and may require oxygen, fluids and steroids to reduce the inflammation. Viral meningitis is usually mild and treated at home with painkillers and anti-emetics (for the sickness). Severe cases will be treated in the same way as bacterial meningitis until it is definitely confirmed to be viral and then the antibiotics withdrawn.

Prognosis: Viral meningitis usually gets better in a few weeks. Bacterial meningitis causes death in about 10% of cases, and complications such as hearing problems are common.

Holistic Advice: Prevention is better than cure and vaccinations are available to help protect against some strains. Boost the immune system.

Menopause

Definition: Cessation of the menstrual cycle.

Possible Causes: Most commonly a natural part of ageing caused by the change in the balance of the sex hormones, specifically oestrogen. Menopause can also be triggered by treatments for breast cancer, chemotherapy, radiotherapy or underlying conditions such as Down's syndrome or Addison's disease. Early or premature menopause can happen at any age and there is often no clear cause.

General Signs and Symptoms: Can occur at any time between the ages of 45 and 55. Periods start to become less frequent over months or years before they stop altogether. Menopause is said to be reached if 12 months pass without a period. Perimenopause begins the transition to menopause and carries additional symptoms that can start up to ten years before menstruation stops. These include hot flushes, night sweats, vaginal dryness, periods of low mood, anxiety, reduced libido (sex drive), difficulty sleeping, headaches, heart palpitations, recurrent urinary tract infections and memory or concentration problems. The severity and duration of these symptoms vary in each individual.

Conventional Medical Treatment: The main treatment for menopausal symptoms is hormone replacement therapy (HRT) which is available in tablets, skin patches, gel (topical) or implants. HRT can be combined (oestrogen and progesterone) or oestrogen only. HRT can help prevent osteoporosis however, the effect does not last long after treatment finishes. Cognitive behavioural therapy (CBT) can be used to help cope with mood swings, low mood or anxiety.

Prognosis: Over time, symptoms should reduce. Menopause can increase the risk of developing osteoporosis (weak bones) due to lack of oestrogen in the body.

Holistic Advice: For hot flushes and night sweats, wear light clothing, reduce stress levels and avoid spicy food, caffeine, smoking and alcohol. Take regular exercise and lose weight if required. To prevent osteoporosis ensure a healthy diet, regular weight bearing exercise, stopping smoking, reducing alcohol and increase vitamin D intake via sunlight or supplements.

Menorrhagia

Definition: Heavier than normal bleeding during menstruation.

Possible Causes: Sometimes the cause is not apparent and, particularly for those who normally have heavy periods, there is probably no need for concern. However, it can be a symptom of uterine disorders such as fibroids, polyps, endometriosis, persistent pelvic infections, polycystic ovary syndrome, or cancer of the uterus, and can also be caused by hormonal disorders such as hypothyroidism. It may be a side effect of using an intrauterine contraceptive device. Risk factors include being over weight, approaching the menopause, anti-coagulant medicines and chemotherapy.

General Signs and Symptoms: Heavy menstrual bleeding which may include blood clots. There may be a dragging pain in the lower abdomen.

Conventional Medical Treatment: Depends on the cause and severity of the condition. A variety of drugs can be prescribed to reduce or stop the bleeding. Depending on the cause, surgical options may be possible. A hysterectomy will stop menstrual bleeding but is only considered as a last resort.

Prognosis: Severe menstrual bleeding, if left untreated, may lead to iron deficiency anaemia.

Holistic Advice: Can cause disruption to many aspects of life style, affecting the woman physically, emotionally and socially.

Migraine

Definition: Intense headache. There are two types – common migraine, which is a severe headache with no warning symptoms, and classical migraine, in which the headache is experienced after warning symptoms (collectively know as the "aura") such as visual disturbances, anxiety, mood swings, changes in energy levels, co-ordination problems, speech difficulties, muscular stiffness or tingling in the neck and shoulders, and an altered sense of taste and smell.

Possible Causes: Thought to be caused by chemical changes in the brain. The aura may be caused by a sudden restriction of blood flow to the brain, and the migraine itself is associated with an increased blood flow. There are many possible trigger factors including hormonal changes associated with menstruation or menopause, anxiety, stress, tension (particularly in the neck and shoulders), shock, depression, excitement, irregular meals, prolonged lack of food, diet, alcohol, over-exertion, physical and mental fatigue, changes of routine, late rising (too much sleep), some medicines, fluorescent lights, flickering screens, changes in weather and sensitivity to certain substances, e.g. paint, petrol, perfume.

General Signs and Symptoms: Commonly a throbbing pain at the front or on one side of the head, worsened by movement. The migraine itself may cause nausea and an increased sensitivity to light, sounds and smells. Body temperature may fluctuate, concentration may be affected, and there may be abdominal pain and a need to urinate frequently. In attacks of classical migraine, the "aura", as described above, is experienced first. Symptoms of migraine can last from a few hours to several days and are more common in women than men.

Conventional Medical Treatment: Painkillers, anti-inflammatory drugs, and anti-sickness medicines are commonly used to ease the symptoms. More specific anti-migraine drugs, such as triptan medicines, may be prescribed. Triptan medicines, if taken at the beginning of an episode or during the aura stage, may prevent the migraine from developing further.

Prognosis: There is no cure but, although they can be disabling, migraine episodes can usually be managed by the effective use of treatments.

Holistic Advice: A regular massage can be a very good preventative treatment to release stress and tension. Keep a diary of food eaten to see if diet is the cause. Cheese, chocolate and red wine are the most common dietary triggers. Eat regularly, follow a regular sleep pattern, and try to reduce stress.

Modified Respiratory Movements

Definition: The muscles of the respiratory system can perform a series of movements as a result of different stimuli. Coughing and hiccoughs are covered elsewhere in this book.

Crying: The shedding of tears in response to emotional state (sadness, anger or happiness), pain or physical irritation of the eye. Characterised by inhalation followed by many short convulsive exhalations.

Laughing: Most commonly an audible expression of positive emotions such as joy, happiness and relief. External stimulus such as being tickled or hearing a funny story can cause laughter. Laughter can also occur with feelings of embarrassment, surprise or nervousness. Much like crying, it is characterised by inhalation followed by short exhalations.

Sighing: Associated with feelings of relief, sadness, exhaustion and stress, sighing can also be used to communicate. Characterised by a long, slow inhalation quickly followed by a shorter more forceful exhalation.

Sneezing: Also known as sternutation, sneezing is the body's way of removing irritants from the nose and throat via a powerful involuntary expulsion of air. Characterised by a long inhalation followed by a single explosive exhalation. Allergens, infections (viruses) and irritants can trigger sneezing.

Talking: Involves using structures of the respiratory system to articulate thoughts and feelings. A deep intake of air supports the voice for speech, allowing the vocal cords to vibrate as air is exhaled.

Yawning: Also known as oscitation, yawning is commonly associated with tiredness, stress, sleepiness and boredom. Yawning can be triggered by seeing or perceiving others yawning and is sometimes coupled with stretching of arms, neck, shoulders and back. Characterised by a deep inhalation through a widely opened mouth.

Motor Neurone Disease

Definition: Progressive degeneration of the nerves in the brain and spinal cord that control muscular activity.

Possible Causes: The motor neurones lose function but the exact cause is unknown. There may be a familial link. There are several types of motor neurone disease. They all have similar symptoms but the speed of progression varies.

General Signs and Symptoms: The motor neurones control voluntary activity such as walking, speaking, breathing and swallowing and so these functions are affected by this condition. Initially sufferers experience muscle weakness, clumsiness, general tiredness, muscle pains, cramps and twitches, and slurred speech. As the condition progresses there is muscle wastage, loss of mobility in the limbs, muscle pain, speech difficulties, drooling, excessive yawning, and problems swallowing. The condition may result in total paralysis and severe breathing difficulties. There may be mood swings and understandably the sufferer often becomes anxious and depressed.

Conventional Medical Treatment: Riluzole is only drug that may directly help the condition but it only gives about another 3 months of life. Other treatments focus on relieving the symptoms both physical and emotional, and so counsellors, physiotherapists and speech therapists may all be involved. A plan will be put in place to ensure the care given when the sufferer can no longer communicate is what was wanted.

Prognosis: It is a rare, serious and incurable disease.

Holistic Advice: Support groups can offer advice and self-help guidance for the sufferer and his/her family.

Mouth Ulcer

Definition: An open sore on the lining of the mouth. The medical name is aphthous ulcer.

Possible Causes: Usually non-infectious and caused as a result of damage to the mouth tissues (e.g. biting the inside of the cheek or rough tooth brushing). Risk factors include stress, anxiety, hormonal changes, certain foods, family history and a depressed immune system. Recurrent mouth ulcers may occasionally be symptomatic of an underlying disease such as iron deficiency, vitamin B_{12} deficiency, folic acid deficiency and some intestinal disorders. Mouth ulcers can also occur as a result of a specific infection such as herpes simplex and pharyngitis.

General Signs and Symptoms: Shallow, grey-white pits with a red border. They can cause pain when eating spicy, hot or acidic foods. Can occur singly or in clusters.

Conventional Medical Treatment: Usually disappear without treatment in a few days. Salty mouth washes may help (don't swallow and seek advice in cases of cardiac problems). Over-the-counter treatments are available.

Prognosis: Usually harmless but consult a Doctor if they do not heal within 3 weeks.

Holistic Advice: To help speed up the healing of a mouth ulcer, use a soft toothbrush, avoid hard foods and try to reduce stress levels.

MRSA

Definition: Abbreviation of methicillin-resistant Staphyloccus aureus, a bacteria that lives on the skin, often harmlessly. It is resistant to many antibiotics and is sometimes referred to as a "superbug".

Possible Causes: MRSA is a common bacterium that lives on the skin often colonising in the nostrils, groin and armpits. The bacteria is transmitted by skin to skin contact with someone who has MRSA, sharing bedding, towels or clothing with someone who has MRSA or touching surfaces/objects that have MRSA on them. People who are staying in hospital are more at risk of contracting MRSA and becoming unwell as a result. This is because they are often in close contact with a large number of people, have inability to fight of the bacteria due to other health issues and often have a way for the bacteria to enter the body such as a wound, drip or catheter.

General Signs and Symptoms: MRSA on the skin does not cause symptoms. If the bacteria is able to enter the skin there may be swelling, pain, pus, redness and swelling in the area. Fever, chills, aches/pains, dizziness and confusion occur if the bacteria goes further into the body.

Conventional Medical Treatment: If found on the body treatment will aim to decolonise the skin of the bacteria. This involves using antibacterial cream inside the nose and washing the skin with antibacterial shampoo. Clothes, towels and bedding will need to be washed every day during treatment. MRSA infection is treated with antibiotics either orally or via injection.

Prognosis: Large majority of cases resolve with treatment. If left untreated MRSA can lead to sepsis which is a serious medical emergency.

Holistic Advice: Maintain good hand hygiene and wound care.

Multiple Sclerosis

Definition: A progressive disease of the brain and spinal cord in which the insulating sheaths of the nerves break up and patches of excessive connective tissue form. Abbreviated to MS.

Possible Causes: MS is an autoimmune disease. It is not known for certain what causes it, but some believe it is caused by a combination of genetic and environmental factors.

General Signs and Symptoms: This condition can have a slow onset and can remit and relapse. The progressive nerve damage affects sensation, movement, body functions and balance. The central nervous system controls the whole body and so, potentially, any part of the body could be affected, but the extent and severity of the symptoms depend on the site and progression of the disease. Numbness and tingling in the extremities commonly occur in the early stages, and in 25% of cases the first symptom is inflammation of the optic nerve, causing visual problems. General weakness and tremors are common upon exertion and sufferers may feel persistent extreme tiredness. There can be muscle spasms causing stiffness, and neuromuscular pain. Speech may become slurred. Problems with co-ordination and cognition may be experienced and it is not uncommon for sufferers to have emotional problems and depression. Stress and heat can worsen the symptoms. MS is the most common nervous system disorder affecting young adults and is twice as likely to affect women than men.

Conventional Medical Treatment: Due to the unpredictability of the condition and the variety of symptoms, care plans will vary. Specialists may be needed to assist mobility, speech, sight, continence and any psychological problems. Drugs to treat some of the symptoms include steroids, painkillers, muscle relaxant drugs, anti-tremor drugs, and antidepressants. Specialist drugs can also be injected to slow the progression of nerve damage.

Prognosis: There is no cure and it is a lifelong condition, but the treatments make it easier to live with. MS does not affect life expectancy but the nerve damage may cause partial paralysis and an affected person may ultimately require a wheelchair for mobility.

Holistic Advice: Take regular, gentle exercise. Yoga can be beneficial to help relaxation as well as stretching the muscles. Reflexology, massage, acupuncture, tia chi and other complementary therapies may help. Minimise stress and avoid high temperatures. There are many support groups for sufferers of MS and their families to get help and advice.

Muscular Dystrophy

Definition: A group of genetic conditions in which muscles become weak and wasted.

Possible Causes: All types of muscular dystrophy are caused by genetic mutations in the genes that control muscular structure and function. The mutations can occur spontaneously but they are usually inherited. Duchenne muscular dystrophy is the most common and the most severe. It affects boys and shows at about the age of 3 years. It begins in the leg muscles before quickly progressing to cause serious disability. Myotonic muscular dystrophy is the most common form in adults. It affects the smaller muscles such as the face, jaws and neck of both sexes.

General Signs and Symptoms: Symptoms vary according to the type of muscular dystrophy and the age of the person when the condition first appeared. For example, in the case of Duchenne muscular dystrophy the legs are first affected so there are problems walking and standing up. The sufferer is usually wheelchair-bound in a few years, develops a curvature (scoliosis) of the spine, has heart problems by the mid-teens, respiratory problems by the late-teens, and is likely to die before the age of 30. In myotonic muscular dystrophy there may be muscle stiffness, cataracts and hormonal problems. The condition is often slow to progress. Some may never progress to serious disability although cardiac problems are possible.

Conventional Medical Treatment: Maintaining mobility for as long as possible is important and so exercise, physiotherapy and physical aids (e.g. braces, crutches and wheelchairs) are used. Some drugs can be used to try to increase muscle strength. Scoliosis of the spine can be corrected by surgery. Cardiac problems can be treated in a variety of ways as and when they occur.

Prognosis: Muscular dystrophy is a progressive disease which becomes life threatening if the cardiac or respiratory muscles are affected. There is no cure but the treatments may help to manage the condition.

Holistic Advice: Support groups can offer advice and self-help guidance for the sufferer and his/her family.

Myalgic Encephalomyelitis

Definition: Abbreviated to M.E., it literally means muscle pain and inflammation of the brain and spinal cord. Also called chronic fatigue syndrome.

Possible Causes: The cause is uncertain, but some think it can be triggered by viral infections that weaken the immune system, e.g. glandular fever, hence it is sometimes referred to as post viral fatigue. Others believe it to be triggered by a combination of physical and psychological factors such as exhaustion, depression, traumatic events, repeated infections, inactivity (or being too active), stress, frustration and poor diet.

General Signs and Symptoms: The main characteristic is generally feeling unwell and extreme fatigue that doesn't decrease with sleep. There are many other possible symptoms including a sore throat, swollen lymph glands, stomach pain, muscle and joint pain (but without inflammation), headaches, intolerance to light, loud noise, alcohol and certain foods, giddiness, palpitations, mood swings, sleeping problems, an inability to concentrate and poor memory. Exercise may worsen the symptoms.

Conventional Medical Treatment: There is no cure, so the treatment focuses on easing the symptoms. The psychological side may be helped by cognitive behavioural therapy to identify thoughts and feelings that trigger behaviour, antidepressants, painkillers, and a tailored exercise programme.

Prognosis: May last for many years. Most cases improve over time enough to resume a normal life, but others continue having symptoms and relapses. Some remain housebound. Early diagnosis, balancing rest with activity, and self help measures can assist.

Holistic Advice: Take plenty of rest and avoid stress of any kind. Maintain a balanced diet. When feeling weak, find an activity that can still be undertaken e.g. a jigsaw. Try relaxation exercises or a massage. Exercise regularly at whatever level can be managed.

Myasthenia Gravis

Definition: Literally means grave muscle weakness. It only affects voluntary muscles.

Possible Causes: Chronic autoimmune disease in which the body produces antibodies that block or damage muscle receptor cells. This causes muscle weakness and excessive muscle fatigue. May be triggered by some viruses or medicines. Genetic make up may also have a role to play although it is not familial.

General Signs and Symptoms: Muscle weakness that gets worse as the day goes on or after activity. Most commonly affects the eye muscles (causing drooping of the eyelid), face and throat muscles (affecting smiling, speech, chewing and swallowing), neck muscles (making it difficult to support the head), and the limbs (creating problems with tasks such as walking upstairs or holding the arms above the head). More rarely, the condition may affect the respiratory muscles, making breathing difficult when exercising or when lying flat. Myasthenia gravis is not usually painful and symptoms that are mild at first get worse over several months.

Conventional Medical Treatment: Cholinesterase inhibitors, to block the action of the chemical that makes muscles relax post-contraction, removal of the thymus gland, which is commonly abnormal in patients with this condition, and steroids and immunosuppressant drugs, to reduce the number of associated antibodies produced, are used to help alleviate symptoms.

Prognosis: No cure but the symptoms can usually be controlled.

Holistic Advice: Try to reduce stress levels and over-exertion. Promote good sleeping habits. The Myasthenia Gravis Association may be able to offer valuable support.

Myositis

Definition: A group of rare autoimmune diseases that causes weak, painful or aching muscles. The two most common types are polymyositis and dermatomyositis.

Possible Causes: Exact cause is unknown. Polymyositis and dermatomyositis are believed to be autoimmune conditions where the body mistakenly attacks its own tissues. Both of the above conditions are more common in women.

General Signs and Symptoms: Polymyositis affects numerous muscles particularly around the neck, shoulders, back hips and thighs. Symptoms include weak, aching and painful muscles, lethargy and fatigue. There may be problems standing or sitting after a fall and difficulty swallowing. The muscles affected by weakness can change week after week and bouts of more intense symptoms are described as a 'flare up'. Dermatomyositis symptoms are similar to polymyositis however there will also be the presence of a rash prior to the muscular symptoms. The rash is usually a distinctive red, purple or dark colour and can be itchy or painful. It commonly appears on the face and hands but can also be seen on the back, chest, elbows and knees. Some people experience symptoms of depression due to this condition.

Conventional Medical Treatment: Treatment is dependent on the type and can be individualised to the person. Steroids are the main medicine used to treat both poly and dermatomyositis by reducing swelling and pain. Disease-modifying anti-rheumatic drugs are a form of immunosuppressant medication that can also help reduce swelling. They can also help reduce the amount of steroid medication needed and reduce the side effects of the steroids. Exercise and physiotherapy are also used to help reduce swelling, build/restore strength and increase energy levels. Speech/language therapy may be recommended to people who have severe myositis if they are finding it hard to speak or swallow.

Prognosis: Most people respond well to a combination of steroids, immunosuppressant medication and exercise. If a person does not respond well to treatment, the condition can have a significant effect on their daily life.

Holistic Advice: Eat a healthy balanced diet and take regular controlled exercise. Build up intensity and duration of exercise gradually. Take regular periods of rest, particularly experiencing a 'flare up'.

Nail Conditions (Additional)

General Information:

Nails may change shape, colour or texture. This is may be due to injury, infection, lifestyle or an underlying disease. Some drugs may also affect the nails.

Minor nail abnormalities that are not associated with underlying disorders, such as white spots caused by minor injury, are unlikely to need treatment. However, if the shape, colour or general condition of the nails changes when no obvious damage has occurred a Doctor should be consulted.

Once the cause of the underlying condition has been treated, the nails should begin to grow normally again. A finger nail can take 6-9 months to grow out and so the process can be slow but the appearance and health of the nails may be improved by having regular manicures or help from a chiropodist.

On the next pages the following other nail conditions will be summarised:

- Beau's Lines
- Brittle Nails
- Discoloured Nails
- Habit Tic
- Hang Nail
- Koilonychia
- Lamellar Dystrophy (Onychoschizia)
- Onychatrophia
- Onychauxis
- Onychogryphosis
- Onychophagy
- Pitting
- Pterygium
- Ridged Nails
- Transverse ridging
- Vertical Streaks

Nail Conditions (Additional) Continued

Beau's Lines: Deep lines or grooves across (side to side) the fingernail. Usually caused by an underlying systemic illness but can also be caused by trauma to the nail.

Brittle Nails: Nails that crack, chip, split or break easily. Often seen due to ageing but can also occur due to frequent exposure to water and detergent. Long-term use of nail polish can also cause brittle nails. Hypothyroidism is a condition that can cause the nails to become brittle.

Discoloured Nails: Nails may become discoloured for many reasons including infection, trauma, lifestyle and an underlying medical disorder. Here are a few examples of the most common causes:
- Yellow nails - infection or heavy smoking
- Green nails - infection
- White nails - nail damage, onycholysis or indicative of liver or kidney disease
- Black nails - collection of blood under the nail from trauma or infection
- Blue nails: may be symptomatic of argyria (caused by the improper exposure to compounds of silver) or Wilson's disease (in which copper builds up in the body) or a lack of oxygen in the blood

Habit Tic: The nail shows damage caused by the habitual picking, scratching or biting of the nail or surrounding tissue.

Hang Nail: Very small pieces of torn skin next to the nail. Commonly caused by trauma such as nail biting or from dry skin.

Koilonychia: Concave spoon-shaped nails. This is usually caused by severe iron deficiency.

Lamellar Dystrophy (Onycoschizia): Horizontal splitting or peeling of the distal end of the nail into layers. Usually caused by water or detergent damage.

Onychatrophia: Permanent atrophy or shrinking of the nail. Most commonly caused by trauma but can also be caused by lichen planus, lupus and scleroderma.

Onychauxis: Thickening of the nail. Can be caused by psoriasis, trauma or fungal nail infections (onychomycosis).

Onychogryphosis: Thickening of the nails. May be due to trauma, neglect or fungal infection. Mostly affects toe nails.

Onychophagy: Clinical name for fingernail biting including the nail plate and sometimes the surrounding tissues of the nail bed and cuticle. Can lead to fungal infections of the nail and surrounding skin.

Pitting: Multiple tiny pits show on the surface of the nail. This is often indicative of an underlying disease such as psoriasis or eczema. It may also be associated with alopecia.

Pterygium: A wing of extra tissue caused by scarring of the nail matrix. Typical of chronic skin condition lichen planus but can also occur due to trauma.

Ridged Nails: The occurrence of longitudinal ridges is normal in the elderly. In younger people it may be indicative of rheumatoid arthritis, lichen planus (a skin condition) and eczema.

Transverse Ridges: Horizontal ridges occurring across the nail. Can occur due to trauma or be a sign of eczema, paronychia and psoriasis.

Vertical Streaks: Vertical streaks are also normal in the elderly and are not usually associated with any underlying disorder.

Nausea

Definition: A feeling of sickness.

Possible Causes: There are many potential causes of nausea. Dizziness from headache, migraine, labyrinthitis or vertigo and infections such as flu can make you feel sick. Morning sickness in early pregnancy can cause nausea. Additionally some medicines and drugs can cause nausea. In some cases, anxiety can make a person feel sick.

General Signs and Symptoms: Feeling like you might, or want to vomit.

Conventional Medical Treatment: Nausea will often not require any medical treatment. If there is a known or suspected underlying cause of the nausea (i.e. infection, food poisoning, headache) treating this may make the feeling go away. If the feeling of nausea persists then anti-sickness medicine can be prescribed.

Prognosis: Feeling sick is very common and often goes away without any medical treatment.

Holistic Advice: Distract yourself from the feeling of nausea and get plenty of fresh air. Try drinking ginger or peppermint tea or taking small sips of a cold drink. Do not cook or eat strong smelling foods and try to eat slowly.

<u>Nephroblastoma (Wilms Tumour)</u>

Definition: Cancer of the kidneys that typically affects children under the age of 5.

Possible Causes: Exact causes are unknown. A small portion of those diagnosed with nephroblastoma will have another condition or congenital abnormality.

General Signs and Symptoms: The most common symptom is a painless mass in the abdomen. Some will also have abdominal pain, hypertension (high blood pressure), fever, blood in the urine, weight loss and anaemia. Nephroblastoma usually only affects one kidney but in rare cases can affect both.

Conventional Medical Treatment: Dependent on the stage and the tumour itself. If possible, the tumour will be removed via surgery. Surgery usually involves removing the entire kidney but in some cases, only part of the kidney will be removed. Chemotherapy and radiotherapy may also be used before and after surgery.

Prognosis: Regular follow-ups will be required to ensure that the cancer has not returned. Very few children suffer long term kidney problems after one of the kidneys are removed. There are chances of some adverse effects from treatment in later years including reduction in bone growth, infertility, problems with heart and lung function and a small chance of developing another cancer. Survival rates are higher for children who only have a tumour in one kidney.

Holistic Advice: If any of the symptoms above are experienced, seek medical advice.

Neuralgia

Definition: Literally means nerve (neur-) pain (-algia). There are 2 main types - trigeminal neuralgia, which is a sudden and severe nerve pain that affects the face for just a few minutes, and postherpetic neuralgia, which is a constant and severe nerve pain brought on by shingles.

Possible Causes: Trigeminal neuralgia is thought to be caused by blood vessels pressing on the root of the trigeminal nerve. It may also be caused by a tumour or multiple sclerosis. Postherpetic neuralgia is caused by the shingles virus. The shingles virus damages the nerves and it is thought that the scar tissue which develops may press on the nerves causing the pain.

General Signs and Symptoms: In trigeminal neuralgia the stabbing, shooting pain is usually felt on only one side of the face, and only for a very short time. The episodes may repeat 100s of times a day or not recur for years. Pain is usually in the jaws, cheek, eye and forehead and may be felt in the mouth. The pain may be triggered by certain actions or movement. Sufferers of postherpetic neuralgia will experience a constant and severe burning, aching or throbbing where the shingles occurred, some stabbing or shooting pain and intense itching.

Conventional Medical Treatment: Anticonvulsants (to prevent seizures) can be effective for trigeminal neuralgia (normal painkillers are not strong enough). Surgery may be necessary. Painkillers, analgesic creams and antidepressants are the most common treatment for postherpetic neuralgia although anticonvulsants may also be used.

Prognosis: Trigeminal neuralgia is a chronic condition that often gets worse over time. Symptoms can be treated but surgery may be required. Postherpetic neuralgia can get better after a few months but can last much longer. Treatment may not completely relieve the pain.

Holistic Advice: For trigeminal neuralgia, avoid wind and draughts, and be wary of eating and drinking hot or cold foods. In cases of posthepetic neuralgia, wear loose fitting clothing and cover sensitive areas to prevent rubbing. Cold packs may help.

Neuritis

Definition: Inflammation of one or more nerves.

Possible Causes: Nerve inflammation can be caused by bacterial infections such as leprosy and Lyme disease. It can also be caused by viral infections such as HIV and the herpes simplex virus. Multiple sclerosis and neuromyelitis optica are both autoimmune diseases that frequently cause optic neuritis (inflammation of the optic nerve). Guillian-Barre syndrome, also an autoimmune condition, can affect the motor nerves causing paralysis. Some forms of cancer can also cause neuritis.

General Signs and Symptoms: Dependent on the location and type of inflamed nerve. Common symptoms experienced are pain, tenderness, impaired sensation, numbness or hypersensitivity, impaired strength, impaired reflexes and abnormal circulation. Inflammation of the optic nerve (optic neuritis) can cause vision disturbances, temporary vision loss and pain when moving the eye. Vestibular neuritis can cause dizziness, vertigo, balance issues and nausea.

Conventional Medical Treatment: Treatment dependent on underlying cause. If caused by bacterial infection, antibiotics can be prescribed. Some episodes of neuritis go away without any medical intervention.

Prognosis: Dependent on the underlying cause.

Holistic Advice: Maintain a healthy balanced diet for general wellbeing.

Non-Hodgkin Lymphoma

Definition: Cancer that develops in the lymphatic system. There are more than 60 types.

Possible Causes: A mutation in a subset of the white blood cells, which causes them to multiply uncontrollably. It can occur at any age, with a third of cases found in the over 75's. Slightly more common in men, it is not clear what triggers or causes this to happen. Risk factors that increase the chance of developing this condition include a weakened immune system from conditions such as HIV, taking immunosuppressant drugs, previous exposure to the Epstein-Barr virus that causes glandular fever, having an autoimmune condition (e.g. lupus or rheumatoid arthritis), H. Pylori infection and coeliac disease.

General Signs and Symptoms: The most common symptom are painless swellings in the neck, armpit or groin. This is caused by excess lymphocytes collecting in the lymph nodes. Symptoms can be location specific such as abdominal pain if the abdomen is affected. Sometimes there will be more generalised symptoms such as night sweats, unexpected weight loss, fever and an itching sensation over the skin.

Conventional Medical Treatment: Often split into low-grade tumours, where the cancer grows slowly, or high-grade tumours, where the cancer grows aggressively. A wait and see approach can be taken for low grade tumours that aren't causing problematic symptoms. A low grade tumour that is causing issues can be treated with chemotherapy, steroids and targeted immunotherapy. High-grade tumours require immediate treatment. Initial treatment can include a course of chemotherapy, targeted immunotherapy followed by radiotherapy. More advanced high grade tumours require intensive chemotherapy. This will be followed up with stem cell or bone marrow transplants. In very few cases, the initial cancer is removed during biopsy and no further treatment is required.

Prognosis: Dependent on the type of Non-Hodgkin lymphoma and the grade. Some people will experience long term problems including a weakened immune system, infertility and secondary cancers. The risk of developing cardiovascular and lung disease increases after having Non-Hodgkin lymphoma.

Holistic Advice: Maintain a healthy weight. Take steps to boost the immune system.

Non-Specific Urethritis

Definition: Inflammation of the urethra not caused by gonorrhoea.

Possible Causes: Non-specific urethritis is the term used when the cause is not known but it has been established that it is NOT caused by gonorrhoea (a sexually transmitted bacterial infection). However, a sexually transmitted disease called chlamydia, caused by the chlamydia trachomatis bacteria, is often responsible for non-specific urethritis. It can also be caused by urinary tract infections and infections from other bacteria or viruses, particularly those that live in the throat, mouth and rectum that find their way into the urethra. Non-specific urethritis can also be caused by damage to the urethra or its irritation by products it may come into contact with.

General Signs and Symptoms: Men may experience a discharge from the penis, pain on urinating, frequent need to urinate, and redness at the opening of the urethra. Mild cases may be asymptomatic. Women only tend to show symptoms if the inflammation spreads to other parts of the pelvis.

Conventional Medical Treatment: Antibiotics are commonly used to treat any bacterial infection.

Prognosis: Can usually be treated effectively but, in women, if the infection spreads it can cause pelvic inflammatory disease which is a serious and painful disorder. In men there is a danger of persistent urethritis. Sexual health clinics will be able to give advice.

Holistic Advice: Practice safe sex to help avoid contracting the condition. If infected, avoid sex altogether until the infection has cleared up completely.

Nosebleed

Definition: Bleeding from the nose. The medical term is epistaxis.

Possible Causes: Commonly occurs spontaneously, particularly in children. In dry environments or during winter months the membranes lining the nose may become dry and cracked causing a bleed. Injury to the nose can also cause bleeding. Other causes include forceful nose-blowing, the presence of a foreign body in the nose, infection of the upper respiratory tract, the use of anticoagulant drugs, hypertension, or an underlying medical condition such as cancer of the nasopharynx.

General Signs and Symptoms: Bleeding from the nose, usually from just one nostril.

Conventional Medical Treatment: Bleeds are usually minor and stop themselves. Putting direct pressure on both sides of the nose to squeeze the nostrils together and holding if for about 20 minutes whilst leaning forward and breathing through the mouth is often successful. Medical attention should be sought if heavy bleeding persists. The focus of the treatment will be on stopping the bleed and finding the cause. Various procedures are available including packing the nose and cauterizing (sealing) the vessel causing the bleed.

Prognosis: Not usually serious but persistent severe bleeds must be investigated.

Holistic Advice: Don't pick the nose or blow it too hard. Protect the nose when playing sport.

Obesity

Definition: An abnormal or excessive body fat accumulation that presents a risk to health.

Possible Causes: Generally, obesity is caused by consuming more calories than are burnt off via physical activity. The excess energy consumed is stored by the body as fat and over time, will lead to obesity. A poor diet is a major contributor to obesity and can include eating large amounts of processed and fast foods, fizzy drinks, fruit juices and alcohol as well as eating portions that are too large. A lack of exercise or physical activity is another factor in weight gain leading to obesity. Certain medications for epilepsy and diabetes can contribute to weight gain. Some health and genetic conditions, such as Prader-Willi syndrome, hypothyroidism (underactive thyroid gland) and Cushing's syndrome, can contribute to weight gain. However, if conditions like hypothyroidism are managed properly with medications, weight gain should not be an issue. Women with a waist circumference of 80cm or more and men with a waist circumference of 94cm or more are more likely to develop obesity related health problems.

General Signs and Symptoms: There are no specific symptoms but signs include an excess accumulation of body fat. Healthy weight for a person's height can be determined by body mass index (BMI), however this is not used to diagnose obesity as very muscular individuals can have a high BMI. A more appropriate measure to determine excess fat may be waist circumference.

Conventional Medical Treatment: There is no quick fix. Eat and maintain a balanced diet and exercise regularly. A weight loss professional such as a dietician can help create a diet than controls the number of calories whilst being nutritious. In some cases, weight loss surgery may be recommended.

Prognosis: Obesity can lead to a number of health conditions affecting the whole body which can range from mild to severe. These include type 2 diabetes, high cholesterol, coronary heart disease, cancer, asthma, high blood pressure, gastro-oesophageal reflux disease (GORD), gallstones, fertility issues, osteoarthritis, sleep apnoea and liver disease.

Holistic Advice: Take regular, moderate intensity exercise. Set realistic goals and commit.

Oesophageal Cancer

Definition: Cancer found anywhere in the oesophagus, also known as the food pipe.

Possible Causes: Exact cause is often unknown but it is more common in males and people aged over 75. Chronic medical conditions such as gastro-oesophageal reflux disease (GORD) and Barrett's oesophagus increase the risk of developing the disease. Lifestyle factors such as being overweight or obese, smoking, alcohol consumption and consistently drinking very hot drinks all increase the risk of developing this cancer.

General Signs and Symptoms: Common symptoms include dysphagia (difficulty swallowing), persistent indigestion, nausea, unexplained weight loss and pain in the throat or being the breastbone. A persistent cough and hoarse voice may also be experienced.

Conventional Medical Treatment: Dependent on the size, type and location of the cancer. If the cancer has not spread surgery may be used to remove part or, in some cases, all of the oesophagus. Chemotherapy and radiotherapy can be used to kill cancer cells and attempt to stop it from coming back.

Prognosis: Dependent on the size, type and location of the cancer. Problems with swallowing can persist and a soft diet approach may be more comfortable. Alternatively, a feeding tube might be more appropriate.

Holistic Advice: Lose weight if required and stop smoking. Limit alcohol consumption and do not drink very hot drinks.

<u>Onychia</u>

Definition: Infection of the nail and nail bed.

Possible Causes: Most often caused by trauma to the nail. Also associated with several conditions including psoriasis, eczema and diabetes.

General Signs and Symptoms: Inflammation, swelling and pain in the affected nail. The nail may become discoloured. Pus may be present and can leak from the nail, increasing the chance of the infection spreading to the surrounding nails and tissues. The nail may become loose and fall off.

Conventional Medical Treatment: Treatment often focuses on the affected part of the nail with some or all off the nail being removed. Drainage of pus from under the nail may be required in some instances. Oral and topical antibiotics may be recommended to treat the infection.

Prognosis: Can be treated but can take several months to resolve fully. If left untreated the infection can spread to other nails.

Holistic Advice: Take care of nails, keep them short and wear appropriate well-fitting footwear. Do not bite the nails or surrounding tissues. Wash the feet regularly and dry them properly. Change socks or tights every day. Boost the immune system.

Onycholysis

Definition: The loosening or separation of a nail from the nail bed.

Possible Causes: Can be caused by damage to the nail and prolonged immersion of the hands in water. Also associated with several conditions including psoriasis, dermatitis, lichen planus of the nail (itchy rash of small, raised, flat-topped lesions that are shiny and pink/purple), certain thyroid problems, bacterial infections and fungal infections. Can be a side effect of some drugs.

General Signs and Symptoms: Opaque or whitened portion on the nail shows the area of separation. The nail may become thicker, pitted and cracked. Separation usually starts at the tip of the nail and works back. The tissues underneath the nail may become infected, making the nail appear green.

Conventional Medical Treatment: When symptomatic of another disease, treating the underlying cause should improve the onycholysis.

Prognosis: Nails grow continually throughout life and so will grow back unless the nail bed is damaged.

Holistic Advice: Take care of nails, keep them short and avoid contact with irritants. When possible, wear gloves to avoid getting the nails wet.

Onychomycosis

Definition: Fungal nail infection.

Possible Causes: Spread of fungal skin infections, such as athlete's foot, to the nail (called tinea unguium). Moist, sweaty feet provide an ideal environment for the growth of fungi. Fingernail infections are often caused by a yeast called candida that can cause infections of the skin around the nails. Damaged skin surrounding the nail is more likely to become infected so those with damaged skin or nails are at greater risk, as are those with a weakened immune system.

General Signs and Symptoms: Thickened, discoloured nail that can turn white, black, yellow or green. Pieces of the brittle nail may fall off or the whole nail can be lost. The underlying and surrounding tissues can become inflamed and painful. Men suffer from onychomycosis more that women and the incidence increases with age.

Conventional Medical Treatment: Mild cases may not need treatment. When treatment is required antifungal tablets and antifungal nail paints can be used.

Prognosis: Can be treated and usually cured but treatment can take several months. If left untreated the infection can spread to other nails.

Holistic Advice: Look after the nails. Do not bite the nails or surrounding tissues. Wash the feet regularly and dry them properly. Change socks or tights every day. Boost the immune system.

Osteo Arthritis

Definition: Arthritis literally means inflammation of a joint. Osteoarthritis is an inflammatory disease of one or more joints in which the cartilage degenerates. There are many types of arthritis but osteoarthritis is the most common. Rheumatoid arthritis is more severe but less common. In rheumatoid arthritis the body's immune system attacks and destroys the joint(s). We'll focus on osteoarthritis, because it affects about 8.5 million people in the UK.

Possible Causes: Cause it not fully known but there may be a genetic predisposition to developing the disease. It is brought on by a reduced ability of the body to repair a joint(s). The cartilage becomes worn and uneven and the bones become thicker and broader, causing stiffness and pain in the affected joint(s). It may be caused by excessive joint usage, congenital bone deformity or simply excessive wear and tear. It can follow injury (e.g. fracture), and can be brought on by other inflammatory diseases. Obesity and repetitive movements may also be triggers.

General Signs and Symptoms: Localized inflammation due to the bones rubbing together. The joints (often the knees, hips and finger joints) may be painful, swollen, stiff (particularly after rest until they get going again) and deformed causing a lack of mobility. Joints may crack and creak, develop bony growths and may also become misaligned.

Conventional Medical Treatment: Variety of painkillers and anti-inflammatory drugs can be used to treat the symptoms. Some painkillers can be applied topically and others (typically corticosteroids) can be injected directly into the joint. In severe instances, and when possible, surgery can be used to restore the cartilage, replace joints (commonly the hip and knee) or to fuse the joints (to make the joint stronger and less painful). Physiotherapy can help joint mobility.

Prognosis: There is no cure for arthritis, but drugs can help reduce the symptoms. Controlling weight, ensuring good posture and avoiding stress and injury to the joints can help. Exercise can help maintain the range of joint movement and strengthen the muscles to better support the joints.

Holistic Advice: Avoid red meats, pork products, tea, coffee and alcohol. The supplements chondroitin and glucosamine are commonly taken. Take gentle exercise. Consider acupuncture and aromatherapy massage. Always treat the whole person. Look at the cause of any stress, any obesity and diet.

Osteogenesis Imperfecta

Definition: Genetic disorder characterised by bones that break easily. Also known as brittle bone disease.

Possible Causes: Caused by a genetic defect that affects the body's ability to make strong bones. This is usually because of a type I collagen deficiency. Type I collagen is normally the most abundant collagen in the body.

General Signs and Symptoms: Bones break easily for little or no obvious reason. Some may experience just a few fractures in a lifetime, others may experience hundreds. It may also cause weak muscles, brittle teeth, a curved spine and hearing loss. There are several types of osteogenesis imperfecta and they are used to categorise the symptoms and severity of the condition.

Conventional Medical Treatment: There is no cure. The treatment focuses on increasing bone mass and muscle strength to help prevent fractures and maintain mobility, as well as controlling the pain associated with fractures. Sufferers are encouraged to exercise as much as possible. Swimming is of particular value as the risk of fracture whilst participating in this form of exercise is small. Walking is also encouraged, even if mobility aids (such as braces and crutches) are required. A surgical procedure called "rodding" can be used, in which metal rods are inserted through the long bones to increase their strength and help prevent and/or correct any deformities.

Prognosis: Depends on the severity of each case.

Holistic Advice: Do everything possible to avoid depleting bone mass by not smoking, and not drinking excess caffeine and alcohol. Eat a balanced, healthy diet and lose any excess weight.

Osteomalacia

Definition: A disorder characterised by weak, soft bones that become distorted or facture easily. In children this condition is called rickets.

Possible Causes: The most common cause of osteomalacia is a deficiency of vitamin D or calcium – both vital for the formation of strong bones. Vitamin D is derived from exposure to sunlight and food such as oily fish, eggs and fortified cereals. Sources of calcium include diary products, green vegetables and wholemeal bread. Children can also be born with a genetic form or rickets, and it can also be caused by underlying conditions that prevent the successful absorption of vitamins and minerals. Risk factors include having a darker skin type (which requires more sunlight for the body to produce sufficient quantities of vitamin D), being born prematurely, and taking medications that affect vitamin D.

General Signs and Symptoms: Rickets can cause bone pain, skeletal deformity, fragile bones that break easily, and dental problems, and it can inhibit growth and development. In adults, symptoms of osteomalacia include waddling when walking, bending bones, muscle weakness and muscle pain.

Conventional Medical Treatment: Rickets and osteomalacia caused by a lack of vitamin D and/or calcium in the diet is treated by dietary supplements, vitamin D injections, and dietary changes to increase the natural intake of vitamin D and calcium. If caused by an underlying medical condition, treating the condition will often help. In cases in which rickets has caused deformities such as bowed legs and curvature of the spine, surgery or the use of braces may be used to correct them, although some deformities may be permanent.

Prognosis: Taking supplements as directed will usually cure the condition although it may take several months before the bone pain and muscle weakness is relieved.

Holistic Advice: Osteomalacia and most cases of rickets can be avoided by ensuring the diet contains sufficient quantities of vitamin D and calcium. Most vitamin D comes from exposure to sunlight and just 15 minutes on the hands a face a few times a week in spring and summer is usually sufficient. Groups at risk of vitamin D deficiency (e.g. the elderly, housebound, those with dark skin and those who do not eat the vitamin D-rich foods) maybe advised to take supplements.

Osteoporosis

Definition: Reduced bone mass and increased porousness of the bone.

Possible Causes: As the body ages, more bone cells are lost than are replaced causing the bones to become thinner and weaker. Osteoporosis therefore develops slowly over several years. Women are at greater risk due to the decrease in oestrogen (essential for healthy bones) levels after the menopause. In men, testosterone helps to maintain healthy bones and so males with a lower level of this hormone may be more susceptible. Osteoporosis is also symptomatic of some diseases such as hyperthyroidism, disease of the renal glands, pituitary gland problems, arthritis, diabetes and renal failure. Lack of calcium salts, low levels of Vitamin D, poor nutrition, heavy drinking, smoking, some drugs and immobilization can also be risk factors. It can be familial.

General Signs and Symptoms: Increased risk of bone fractures. Often breaking a bone under circumstances which would not normally cause a fracture is the first sign of the condition, and tests carried out then result in the diagnosis. It can cause spinal crush, causing pain and loss of height.

Conventional Medical Treatment: Hormone replacement therapy may be recommended to increase the oestrogen level in woman, and men can be given testosterone treatment. Calcitonin can be given to inhibit the cells that break down bone. Other drugs can be used to help maintain bone density, and calcium and vitamin D supplements may be prescribed.

Prognosis: The body, particularly in the elderly, may not be able to heal the fractures effectively, so it can cause long term issues. As the bones weaken and give way, the condition itself may increase the likelihood of falls, so exacerbating the problem.

Holistic Advice: Seek nutritional advice regarding supplements and dairy intake. Maintain a healthy diet that contains calcium, stop smoking and limit alcohol intake. Regular exercise, including weight-bearing exercises, can help maintain bone strength and help prevent this condition.

Ovarian Cysts

Definition: A fluid filled sac that develops on the ovary. Can be categorised as functional or pathological.

Possible Causes: Functional ovarian cysts develop naturally and are linked to the menstrual cycle. They are non-cancerous and often harmless, disappearing after a few months without treatment. Pathological cysts are caused by abnormal cell growth and are not related to the menstrual cycle. They develop both before and after menopause and can grow so large that they block the blood supply to the ovaries. Endometriosis and polycystic ovary syndrome (PCOS) are two conditions that can cause ovarian cysts.

General Signs and Symptoms: Very common and often do not cause any symptoms. Symptoms usually only occur if the cyst is very large, blocks blood supply to the ovaries or ruptures. These symptoms include dull to severe pelvic pain, pain during sex, frequent urination, irregular periods, bloating, difficulty emptying the bowels and feeling full after eating very little.

Conventional Medical Treatment: In the majority of cases an ultrasound scan will be done a few weeks or months after initial diagnosis to see if the cyst is still present. If it has gone, no further treatment will be needed. If treatment is required it will depend on the size, appearance, symptoms experienced and if the person has been through the menopause. For larger cysts that have potential to be or become cancerous, surgery under general anaesthetic is recommended.

Prognosis: As majority of ovarian cysts go away in a few months, the outcome is very good. If post-menopausal there is a slightly higher chance of developing ovarian cancer so regular monitoring will be required. If surgery is needed there will be a recovery period which may last up to 12 weeks. Fertility will be preserved where possible. Complications such as heavy bleeding, pain in the abdomen and fever can be associated with infection after surgery.

Holistic Advice: If any symptoms are noticed, make an appointment with the GP.

Paget's Disease Of The Bone

Definition: A condition that affects the cycle of bone renewal.

Possible Causes: Exact cause is unknown. Osteoclasts (cells that absorb old bone) begin to absorb bone at a faster rate than normal. The osteoblasts (cells that create new bone) attempt to compensate by producing new bone faster but this results in weak bone formation.

General Signs and Symptoms: In many cases, there are no symptoms. Can affect singular or many bones at the same time, anywhere in the body. Common areas affected are the pelvis, shoulders, legs, spine and skull. Symptoms can include constant, dull bone pain which is worse at night. Swelling, stiffness and pain in the joints can be caused by abnormal bone growth damaging nearby cartilage. In some instances nerves can be compressed by abnormal bone growth leading to numbness, tingling and loss of movement.

Conventional Medical Treatment: Treatment aims to relieve symptoms. Painkillers can be used to treat pain. Bisphosphonate medication be prescribed to control bone regeneration. Vitamin D and calcium supplements may be prescribed. Assistance devices such as walking sticks and shoe inserts can be beneficial. Surgery may be required to correct fractures, deformities or joint damage.

Prognosis: There is no cure but treatment can help improve symptoms. Complications can include fragile bones that break easily, enlarged bones and too much calcium in the blood. Hearing loss can occur if the skull is affected. In rare cases bone cancer can develop.

Holistic Advice: Bone strength can be helped by ensuring a balanced diet that includes calcium. Good sources of calcium include milk, cheese, yoghurt and green leafy vegetables. Vitamin D, formed naturally by the skin when exposed to sunlight, helps the body to absorb calcium. Vitamin D is also found in eggs and oily fish.

Pancreatic Cancer

Definition: Cancer found anywhere in the pancreas.

Possible Causes: Exact cause is not always known. Pancreatic cancer is much more common in people aged 75 and over. Conditions such as pancreatitis, diabetes and gallstones are risk factors for pancreatic cancer. Lifestyle factors that increase risk of developing this disease include smoking, heavy alcohol consumption and being overweight or obese. Pancreatic cancer has been shown to run in families.

General Signs and Symptoms: Symptoms may be non-existent or non-specific making them difficult to identify. Common symptoms include pain in the stomach or back, jaundice and unexplained weight loss. Further symptoms include nausea, vomiting, indigestion, feeling bloated, changes in bowel habits, fever and fatigue.

Conventional Medical Treatment: Treatment dependent on location, size and type of cancer. If it is found early enough surgery can be used to remove the cancer. Surgery can also be used to help control symptoms if the cancer cannot be removed. Chemotherapy and radiotherapy can also be used to kill the cancer cells and try to prevent them returning in the future.

Prognosis: Dependent on location, size and type of cancer. Enzyme supplements may be required to aid digestion after surgery if the pancreas is no longer functioning properly. Blood sugar will also regulated via insulin or medication after surgery. Painkillers and/or nerve blockers may be required to control pain from the disease.

Holistic Advice: Stop smoking, reduce alcohol consumption and lose weight if required.

Parkinson's Disease

Definition: A progressive brain disorder characterized by tremors, rigidity and impairment of voluntary movement.

Possible Causes: Parkinson's disease is characterised by low levels of the neurotransmitter dopamine. The reduction of the dopamine level is due to the loss of nerve cells in a part of the brain called the substantia nigra that are responsible for producing dopamine. The correct balance of dopamine and another neurotransmitter called acetylcholine is necessary for fine muscle control and smooth movement. It is not known why these brain cells are lost but it may be due to genetic and/or environmental factors.

General Signs and Symptoms: Slowness of movement, lack of co-ordination, difficulty with fine movements, tremors and muscle rigidity are the most typical symptoms. In the early signs the tremors tend to affect only one hand, arm or leg, usually at rest, and then later both sides are affected. The face may also lose its natural movement and the voice may alter due to the muscles of the larynx, tongue and lips changing. Speech may become impaired and there may be difficultly swallowing. Sufferers may also suffer from tiredness, depression and continence problems. The symptoms usually begin slowly and then gradually develop but in no particular order. Parkinson's affects everybody differently. It is more common in men than women, and is more likely after the age of 60.

Conventional Medical Treatment: Various drugs can be used to try to balance the levels of neurotransmitters in the brain to help relieve the symptoms. Anticholinergic drugs (given to help reduce muscular spasms) may also help reduce shaking and stiffness. Specialists may be needed to assist mobility, speech, continence and any psychological problems. Surgery is occasionally used on young suffers.

Prognosis: There is no cure. The treatments are available to help control the symptoms but cannot change the progression of the disease. Although many can lead an active life for many years after diagnosis, most will eventually need daily help and symptoms may get harder to treat.

Holistic Advice: Yoga can be beneficial to counteract the stiffening process. Promote a regular sleeping pattern, take regular exercise and maintain a healthy diet. Help groups can give valuable support and advice.

Paronychia

Definition: Infection of the fold of skin that surrounds a nail.

Possible Causes: Acute paronychia comes on quickly and is caused by a bacterial infection that enters the body through a cut or break in the skin that makes up the nail fold. Biting the nails can therefore make infection more likely. Those with decreased resistance to infection due to other underlying conditions are more susceptible. Chronic paronychia can develop over months and is common in those who have their hands in water for prolonged periods. The skin around the nail separates from the nail, softens, and then becomes infected usually by a yeast organism.

General Signs and Symptoms: Pain, swelling and redness in the infected area. The swelling may be filled with pus. Infection can spread to the fingertip causing finger pulp infection. If left untreated the nail may separate from the nail bed.

Conventional Medical Treatment: Antibiotics or antifungal drugs to treat the infection. Pus filled swellings may need to be drained.

Prognosis: Usually clears up quickly with treatment.

Holistic Advice: Anything to boost the immune system will help. Keep hands dry when possible, and maintain good hand hygiene.

Pediculosis

Definition: Infestation of lice. Three types of lice can infest humans namely, pediculus humanus capitis (head lice), pediculus humanus corporis (body lice) and phthirus pubis (pubic lice).

Possible Causes: Head lice infestation (pediculosis capitis) occurs through via head to head contact. They live on the scalp and hair and is the most common of the three. Body lice infestation (pediculosis corporis) occurs when there is very close contact or sharing of bedding/clothing with an infected person. They live on clothing and move to the body to feed. They are more common in crowded living situations and areas of extreme poverty. Public lice infestation (pediculosis pubis) are transmitted by close or sexual contact. They often live in the pubic hair but can spread to the eyelashes, armpit, beard and chest hair.

General Signs and Symptoms: The main symptom for all three infestations is itching. There may be sensations of the lice moving across the infested area or sightings of live lice. Blood spots on the underclothing may be present in pubic lice infestation.

Conventional Medical Treatment: Head and pubic lice can both be treated with insecticides. Head lice can also be removed using a fine toothed detection comb. Body lice is treated by laundering clothing on a hot wash and tumble dry.

Prognosis: Head lice do not carry any other infectious diseases but infestation is very hard to prevent. Complications from pubic lice come from itching, which can increase the risk of bacterial infection. Body lice can transmit other diseases.

Holistic Advice: Treat immediately following detection. Good personal hygiene practices are important to prevent body lice.

Pelvic Inflammatory Disease (PID)

Definition: Infection of the female upper genital tract, which can include the womb, fallopian tubes and ovaries.

Possible Causes: Large majority of cases are caused by bacterial infection. Often these bacteria come from a sexually transmitted infection (STI) such a chlamydia, gonorrhoea or mycoplasma genitalium. If not caused by an STI, it will be caused by bacteria that are normally found in the vagina which make their way into past the cervix. This is more likely to happen if there has been previous instance of pelvic inflammatory disease, damage to the cervix following childbirth or miscarriage or previous procedures that have opened the cervix.

General Signs and Symptoms: Often no obvious symptoms. Can cause one or more of the following; lower abdominal pain, discomfort/pain during sex felt deep in the pelvis, pain on urination, bleeding between periods or after sex, heavy and painful periods. On rare occasions, the pain in the abdomen can be severe with fever and vomiting.

Conventional Medical Treatment: If caught early it can be treated easily and effectively with a course of antibiotics. Any sexual partners within 6 months of treatment will also need to be tested and treated.

Prognosis: Complications of delayed treatment or repeat infections can include scarred and narrowed fallopian tubes, causing fertility issues as well as ectopic pregnancies. Abscesses can also develop on the fallopian tubes and ovaries. In some cases, chronic pelvic pain can occur.

Holistic Advice: As PID is often caused by STI, use of a condom or barrier during sexual intercourse or oral sex is recommended to prevent infection. Do not share sex toys.

Peptic Ulcers

Definition: An open sore on the lining of the oesophagus (oesophageal ulcer), stomach (gastric ulcer) or on the lining of the first part of the small intestine (duodenal ulcer).

Possible Causes: The majority of peptic ulcers are due to an infection by the Helicobacter pylori (H. pylori) bacteria. These bacteria damage the protective mucus lining of the oesophagus, stomach and small intestine, leaving the underlying tissue subject to erosion by the acidic digestive juices. This allows open sores to form. Peptic ulcers can also be caused by the long term use of some drugs such as aspirin and ibuprofen, which damage the stomach lining. Risk factors include age, family history, smoking, and alcohol consumption.

General Signs and Symptoms: The most common symptom is burning pain or discomfort in the upper abdomen. There may also be loss of appetite, weight loss, a feeling of fullness in the abdomen, nausea and sometimes vomiting. Pain may be worse before meals when the stomach is empty. When the ulcer is in the oesophagus there can be lower chest pain and difficulty swallowing. Stress may worsen symptoms.

Conventional Medical Treatment: Antibiotics can be used if the condition is caused by a bacterial infection. Antacids can help relieve the symptoms and a variety of drugs are available to help reduce acidity, giving the ulcers time to heal. If the ulcers are caused by medication, a change of drugs will be considered. Tests may be carried out to rule out more serious conditions.

Prognosis: If treatment is received, the outcome is usually very good. Without treatment the ulcer may bleed, causing a loss of blood, or the ulcer may perforate through the wall of the digestive tract allowing its contents into the abdomen. This can cause peritonitis (inflammation of the lining of the abdomen) and can be fatal. The inflammation may also cause gastric obstruction

Holistic Advice: Make lifestyle changes to reduce stress. Cut down on alcohol and caffeine and stop smoking. Boost the immune system to help protect against infection.

Peripheral Neuropathy

Definition: An umbrella term for a group of conditions where the peripheral nervous system is damaged. The main types are sensory, motor, autonomic and mononeuropathy.

Possible Causes: Occurs when the nerves in the extremities are damaged (e.g. the hands, feet, arms). Diabetes is the most common cause of peripheral neuropathy (known as diabetic polyneuropathy). The risk of developing diabetic polyneuropathy increases if blood sugar is poorly controlled, the person smokes, drinks alcohol excessively or is over 40 years old. Other health conditions that cause peripheral neuropathy are vitamin B12 deficiency, hypothyroidism, lymphoma, multiple myeloma, chronic liver or kidney disease and inflammation of the blood vessels. Infections such as shingles, Lyme disease, diphtheria and HIV can also cause peripheral neuropathy. Chemotherapy, some antibiotics and epilepsy medication can also cause this condition. Chronic excessive alcohol consumption increases the risk of developing peripheral neuropathy.

General Signs and Symptoms: Dependent on which nerves are affected. Sensory neuropathy symptoms can include pins and needles, numbness, reduced sense of pain or temperature change, sharp/burning pain and loss of balance/coordination due to lowered ability to tell the position of the hands/feet. Motor neuropathy symptoms can include twitching, cramping, weakness, paralysis and wasting of the muscles. Autonomic neuropathy symptoms include constipation or diarrhoea, nausea, bloating, hypotension, rapid heart beat, problems with sweating, problems with sexual function and difficulty passing urine. Mononeuropathy (e.g. carpal tunnel syndrome) can include altered sensation in the fingers, feet or shins, double vision and Bell's palsy.

Conventional Medical Treatment: Treatment often targets the underlying cause. For example, gain control of diabetes, stopping smoking or maintaining a healthy diet. If a vitamin B12 deficiency is the cause, supplements will be recommended. Medication causing peripheral neuropathy should be stopped if possible. Less commonly steroids, immunosuppressant and injections of immunoglobin may be prescribed. Neuropathic pain medication or strong prescription painkillers may be given if the pain is particularly bad.

Prognosis: Dependent on the underlying cause of the neuropathy. Common in diabetic polyneuropathy is diabetic foot ulcers where numbness on the feet allows a small wound to develop into an ulcer. This can progress to gangrene if left untreated, which can require a toe or foot to be amputated.

Holistic Advice: Stop smoking and limit alcohol consumption. Exercise regularly and eat a healthy balanced diet. Take steps to properly manage diabetes.

Pernicious Anaemia

Definition: Anaemia is the term used to describe disorders in which the haemoglobin in the red blood cells is deficient or abnormal. Pernicious anaemia is an autoimmune disease that affects the stomach, preventing the absorption of vitamin B_{12}. Vitamin B_{12} is one of the necessary components required to produce healthy red blood cells.

Possible Causes: Vitamin B_{12} can only be absorbed from ingested food if it combines with a chemical called the intrinsic factor, which is produced by cells in the stomach. This autoimmune condition attacks the stomach cells, effectively stopping them from secreting the intrinsic factor. This leads to a deficiency in vitamin B_{12} and, as a result, the body produces abnormally large red blood cells that are unable to transport sufficient oxygen to the tissues. Risk factors include being female, being over 60, family history and having another autoimmune disorder. Pernicious anaemia is just one cause of vitamin B_{12} deficiency anaemia.

General Signs and Symptoms: General symptoms of anaemia include tiredness, lethargy, weakness, shortness of breath, palpitations, headache and faintness. Anaemia caused by vitamin B_{12} deficiency also has symptoms including jaundice, loss of balance, disturbed vision and an altered sense of touch. It can also have psychological effects.

Conventional Medical Treatment: Vitamin B_{12} levels can be boosted by regular injections. This will be a lifelong treatment.

Prognosis: Complications are rare but a long-term deficiency of vitamin B_{12} can cause problems.

Holistic Advice: Increasing the vitamin B_{12} in the diet has no effect, but eating a healthy, balanced diet can help ensure the sufficient supply of other vital vitamins.

Pertussis

Definition: Infection of the lining of the airways that causes bouts of coughing. Commonly called whooping cough.

Possible Causes: Caused by the Bordetella pertussis bacteria, which infect the trachea and the bronchi. The infection is highly infectious and transmitted in airborne droplets produced when infected people cough and sneeze.

General Signs and Symptoms: Typified by violent fits of coughing that end in a "whoop" when the person inhales. The symptoms may take up to 20 days to appear after infection. The symptoms resemble the common cold at first, and then worsen and the "whooping" cough develops. This may be accompanied by the production of large amounts of sputum. The severe coughing may cause vomiting and the rupture of small blood vessels, resulting in a rash of small, flat, red spots, especially around the face, hairline and eyes. The coughing can be very tiring, particularly for young children. Whooping cough usually affects infants and young children although adults can be affected.

Conventional Medical Treatment: The infection is treated with antibiotics. Seriously ill children may require hospitalisation. The pertussis vaccine is usually given routinely in childhood to protect from this condition.

Prognosis: Most make a full recovery but it can be life threatening in the very young.

Holistic Advice: The infection is highly infectious so great care must be taken not to spread the disease. Take plenty of rest and drink plenty of fluids.

Pharyngitis

Definition: Inflammation of the pharynx (throat), often described simply as a sore throat.

Possible Causes: Commonly caused by a viral infection, such as the common cold, or by a bacterial infection, such as the streptococcal bacteria. Smoking and alcohol may cause the throat to become sore, and a sore throat is sometimes symptomatic of another disease.

General Signs and Symptoms: The sore throat is usually accompanied by difficulty swallowing, swollen tonsils, enlarged neck glands, runny nose, headache, muscle aches and a cough.

Conventional Medical Treatment: Painkillers can help relieve the symptoms, as can throat lozenges containing local anaesthetic.

Prognosis: Pharyngitis usually clears up without treatment within 3-7 days. In severe cases it may cause breathing difficulties. It can develop into a more serious condition if the immune system is compromised.

Holistic Advice: Eating ice cream can help sooth the soreness. Drinking plenty of hot or very cold fluids can help. Hot lemon and honey drinks are good soothers. Using a humidifier to keep the surrounding air moist can be useful. Boost the immune system.

Pleurisy

Definition: Inflammation of the pleura.

Possible Causes: The two pleural membranes, which cover the lungs and separate the lungs from the chest wall, usually slide over each other to allow the lungs to inflate and deflate smoothly. Inflammation prevents this, and they rub together. The resulting friction causes sharp, severe chest pain when inhaling. Can be caused by a viral illness (e.g. flu), autoimmune disorders (e.g. rheumatoid arthritis) and injury to the ribs. Lung damage beneath the pleura, caused by conditions such as pneumonia, pulmonary embolism and lung cancer, can also cause the pleura to become inflamed.

General Signs and Symptoms: Sharp chest pain when inhaling deeply, coughing or sneezing (possibly restricted to just one side depending on the location of the pleurisy). There may be difficulty in breathing and a dry cough. The presence of a fever, a productive cough, serious breathing difficulties or a swollen arm or leg, may indicate a serious underlying condition for which medical attention should be sought quickly. When caused by infection or a pulmonary embolism, the symptoms can have a fast onset. In other cases the symptoms may occur gradually.

Conventional Medical Treatment: Non-steroidal anti-inflammatory drugs to relieve the pain and inflammation. Treatment will also be required for any underlying medical condition.

Prognosis: The condition generally clears up within 7-10 days of the start of treatment.

Holistic Advice: Holding the affected side during coughing may help ease the pain.

Pneumonia

Definition: Inflammation of the lung tissue in one or both lungs.

Possible Causes: The alveoli become inflamed and fill with fluid. This makes it difficult for oxygen to pass into the bloodstream. Inflammation is usually caused by bacterial infection, most commonly Streptococcus pneumoniae, but can be caused by other organisms including viruses and, more rarely, fungi. It can also be caused by breathing something into the lungs that causes an irritation, e.g. vomit, food, smoke or chemicals. There is an increased risk of developing this condition if the immune system is compromised, and those who are already seriously ill, malnourished, smoke or abuse alcohol are also more vulnerable. Legionnaires' disease is a form of pneumonia. It is caused by bacteria that are spread through air-conditioning systems.

General Signs and Symptoms: Pneumonia is typified by a cough that may be dry, but if productive produces thick yellow, green, brown or blood-stained mucus. There may be chest pain that is worse on inhalation, shortness of breath at rest, rapid heartbeat, fever, sweating, shivering and loss of appetite. The symptoms may have a fast or gradual onset depending on the cause.

Conventional Medical Treatment: If caused by a bacterial infection, antibiotics can be prescribed. Painkillers may help the pain and reduce any fever. For mild viral pneumonia no drug treatment is usually required. For severe infections, hospitalization may be necessary.

Prognosis: Although mild cases can usually be treated successfully at home, pneumonia can be fatal, particularly in infants and the elderly. Increasing resistance of some organisms to antibiotics is making some forms of pneumonia harder to treat.

Holistic Advice: Stop smoking. Drink plenty of fluids. Warm lemon and honey drinks may help ease the discomfort caused by coughing. Higher risk groups can be vaccinated against this condition.

Pneumothorax

Definition: When air leaks into the space between the lung and the ribcage. The medical term for collapsed lung.

Possible Causes: Can be spontaneous or traumatic. Spontaneous pneumothorax is further divided into primary and secondary. Primary spontaneous occurs in an otherwise healthy person and there is no apparent cause. Risk factors that increase the chances of this happening are smoking, being tall and thin as well as being male. Secondary spontaneous is when a pneumothorax develops in someone who already has a lung condition, most commonly COPD (chronic obstructive pulmonary disorder). This is because the lung tissue is already damaged, making it weak. Tuberculosis, sarcoidosis, cystic fibrosis and lung cancer are other conditions that can increase the risk of secondary spontaneous pneumothorax. Traumatic pneumothorax can be caused by injury to the chest such as in a car accident. Trauma from surgery or treatment for conditions such as emphysema can also cause traumatic pneumothorax. Previous history of pneumothorax increases the chances of reoccurrence.

General Signs and Symptoms: A small pneumothorax may cause no symptoms. With larger pneumothorax, the air in the space can squash or collapse the lung Symptoms will come on suddenly and include a sharp, stabbing pain on one side of the chest. Breathlessness is also common.

Conventional Medical Treatment: Dependent on the cause and the size. The main aim is to reduce the pressure on the lung and allow it to re-expand. If small, it will usually heal by itself and the trapped air will be reabsorbed by the body. Painkillers can be taken to reduce any pain. If large, aspiration may be performed to suck the air out of the space. Alternatively, a chest drain may be performed by inserting a plastic tube into the chest wall to allow the lung to inflate. Any breathlessness can be treated by giving oxygen. Reoccurring pneumothorax in the same side can be treated by an operation to seal the weak areas of the lung or to permanently stick the outside of the lung to the chest wall (pleurodesis).

Prognosis: Dependent on the cause.

Holistic Advice: Stop smoking.

Poliomyelitis

Definition: Highly infectious disease that can attack the nerves which may lead to muscle paralysis. Poliomyelitis has been eradicated in the UK but remains a serious problem in India, Pakistan, Afghanistan and Nigeria. It is often simply referred to as polio.

Possible Causes: Caused by a virus called enterovirus. It thrives in the gastrointestinal tract and then may move to the nervous system. It is spread by oral contact with faeces from an infected person, commonly through contaminated water and food.

General Signs and Symptoms: For most it is asymptomatic, or only results in a mild illness with a slight fever, sore throat, nausea, vomiting, diarrhoea and constipation. In less than 1%, paralysis may result. The first symptoms of the paralytic form include fever, headache, back and neck stiffness, constipation and increased sensitivity to touch. The damage to the nerve cells leads to muscle weakness, and the limbs may become loose and floppy. Difficulties may be experienced with the senses (sight, sound, smell, taste and touch) and the heart muscle and respiratory muscles may also be affected.

Conventional Medical Treatment: There is no cure and so vaccination is very important to prevent the disease. The treatment can only help to ease the symptoms experienced. Mild cases may be treated with rest and painkillers. Physiotherapy may help speed recovery if the muscles have been affected. Severe cases may require a ventilator to assist breathing.

Prognosis: Most make a full recovery from mild forms of the disease. Many of those who become paralysed improve within 6 months, but some can be left with permanent paralysis and deformity. It has been found that a large percentage of those who contracted polio suffer from post-polio syndrome many years after the infection. Symptoms of post-polio syndrome include fatigue, muscle weakness and muscle and joint pain.

Holistic Advice: Ensure vaccines are up to date before travelling to parts of the world where poliomyelitis is still a risk. A booster may be required.

__Polycystic Ovary Syndrome__

Definition: Multiple, small, fluid-filled follicles in the ovaries.

Possible Causes: The cause in unknown but it is associated with resistance to insulin and sex hormone imbalance. Resistance to insulin causes more to be produced. This increased level of insulin causes the ovaries to produce too much testosterone which interferes with the development of the follicle, prevents normal ovulation and may create "masculine" symptoms such as the increased growth of body hair. It also causes weight gain. Many women with this condition have raised levels in luteinising hormone, follicle stimulating hormone and prolactin, and lower levels of thyroid hormones. This condition tends to run in families and there are connections to a family history of diabetes and high cholesterol. Obesity is a major risk factor.

General Signs and Symptoms: The condition may cause irregular ovulation or prevent it altogether. Sufferers may experience irregular or light periods and infertility problems. Other possible symptoms include the excessive growth of body hair, acne, depression and weight gain. Symptoms may vary in severity and the condition may go unnoticed until tests are carried out to explain the cause of infertility.

Conventional Medical Treatment: The treatment depends on the severity of the symptoms and if the woman wants to conceive. Lifestyles changes can significantly help, particularly losing excess weight. Hormone treatment can be given to reduce testosterone levels which helps to regulate periods and reduce the "maleness" symptoms. Creams can also be used to slow down hair growth. Diabetes drugs can help to treat the insulin resistance and increase ovulation. Fertility drugs can promote fertility. A surgical procedure can use heat or laser on the ovaries to destroy the tissue that is creating the male hormones. Topical treatments can be used to help relieve the symptom of acne.

Prognosis: Cannot be cured but the symptoms can be treated and fertility improved. Left untreated it can lead to type 2 diabetes mellitus, hypertension and high cholesterol levels. There is a greater risk of endometrial cancer in those who have not regularly menstruated for many years.

Holistic Advice: Lose excess weight and exercise regularly. Ensure a healthy balanced diet.

Postnatal Depression

Definition: Depressive feelings or psychological disturbances in the first few weeks or months after childbirth.

Possible Causes: Depression is often triggered by emotional and stressful events. Childbirth tends to be both of these. Postnatal depression was thought to be caused by a fall in hormone levels but now it is thought likely to be caused by a combination of environmental, psychological, physical and emotional factors. Risk factors include previous experiences of depression, family history, feelings of inadequacy and isolation, concerns about new responsibilities, lack of support, relationship or financial worries, lack of sleep, stress, a difficult labour, and physical problems post-birth.

General Signs and Symptoms: The usual symptoms of depression are commonly present, e.g. low self esteem, tearfulness and feelings of despair. The sufferer may feel unable to cope, have panic attacks and dramatic mood swings, experience a lack of motivation and lack of interest in anything (including the baby), and be tired and irritable. Some women also get thoughts about harming their baby.

Conventional Medical Treatment: The earlier the condition is recognized the better. Just admitting to the feelings and talking about them can help. Antidepressants may be prescribed and counselling may be recommended. In very severe cases, where it is thought the baby or mother may be at risk from harm, hospitalisation or admission to a mental health clinic may be required. Electroconvulsive therapy may be recommended if all other treatments have failed.

Prognosis: As long as it is recognised and treated, it is a short-term condition from which a full recovery can be made.

Holistic Advice: Get as much rest and relaxation as possible, take gentle, regular exercise, eat regular, healthy meals, avoid alcohol and talk about feelings. Local support groups can offer help.

Pre-eclampsia

Definition: A condition that affects pregnant women, most commonly after 20 weeks, or soon after the baby is delivered.

Possible Causes: The exact cause is unknown but it is thought that a problem with the placenta causes the condition. Risk factors that increase the chance of pre-eclampsia include, expecting multiple babies (twins or more), being over 40, family history of the condition, being obese, having diabetes, high blood pressure or kidney disease before becoming pregnant. Having other conditions such as lupus or having developed pre-eclampsia in a previous pregnancy also increase chances of it developing.

General Signs and Symptoms: Early signs include hypertension (high blood pressure) and proteinuria (protein in the urine). In some cases fluid retention causing swelling of the feet, ankles and hands. Headache and vision problems can also be experienced.

Conventional Medical Treatment: If a person is thought to be at risk of developing the condition, a daily low-dose of aspirin may be advised from the 12th week of pregnancy. If diagnosed, the condition will be monitored to determine the severity and sometimes medication to control blood pressure will be prescribed. To cure pre-eclampsia, the baby must be delivered and labour may be artificially induced.

Prognosis: Most cases cause no problems. If not treated it can cause serious complications to the mother including convulsions, stroke and HELLP syndrome (liver and bloody clotting disorder). The baby may have slow growth and be delivered before it has fully developed.

Holistic Advice: Minimise risk factors by maintaining a healthy weight and managing any pre-existing conditions.

Premenstrual Syndrome

Definition: Various symptoms that may affect women in the days leading up to menstruation.

Possible Causes: The exact cause is unknown, but it is thought to be due to hormonal and chemical changes associated with menstruation. A chemical called serotonin, known to regulate mood, fluctuates during the menstrual cycle. Low levels may contribute to tiredness, food cravings and insomnia. Risk factors may include being overweight, stress, caffeine, alcohol and chocolate.

General Signs and Symptoms: Vary between women and may change month to month. Symptoms can be physical (e.g. fluid retention, bloating, breast tenderness, abdominal pain, tiredness, headaches or migraine, backache and muscle stiffness), psychological (e.g. mood swings, feeling irritable, depression and difficulty concentrating) and behavioural (e.g. loss of interest in sex and changes in appetite).

Conventional Medical Treatment: Self help measures are encouraged to ensure diet and the level of exercise taken are optimized to reduce risk factors. Failing that, medications such as non-steroidal anti-inflammatories (to ease sore breasts, headaches and muscular pain), diuretic drugs (to reduce water retention and bloating), oral contraceptives and synthetic hormones (to help regulate hormonal activity) and some antidepressant drugs (to help with the psychological effects) can be prescribed. If many symptoms are psychological, therapies such as cognitive behavioural therapy may also be of use.

Prognosis: There is no cure but treatments help the symptoms to be managed.

Holistic Advice: Any therapy that can help reduce stress and promote relaxation may be of benefit. Some find supplements of evening primrose oil and vitamin B6 (very high doses can be harmful) may help. Chamomile tea is calming and diuretic which can help relieve the water retention. Maintain a good, balanced, high fibre, fresh food diet, cutting down on saturated fats, sugar, salt and caffeine. Take regular exercise and try to stay stress free.

Pressure Sore

Definition: An injury to the skin and underlying tissues primarily caused by prolonged pressure on the area. Also known as bed sores or pressure ulcers.

Possible Causes: Pressure sores are caused by a lack of blood flow due to an area of skin that has been under prolonged pressure. They can occur anywhere on the body but are most common over bony areas such as the base of the spine, hips, elbows and heels. Pressure sores are more common in people older people, particularly those who are immobile (e.g. confined to bed due to illness or injury) or sat in a chair or wheelchair for prolonged periods. Conditions that affect blood supply or increase fragility of the skin such as diabetes, peripheral arterial disease, kidney failure, heart failure, multiple sclerosis and Parkinson's disease all increase the risk of developing pressure sores. Smoking, poor diet and obesity are also linked to pressure sores.

General Signs and Symptoms: Often develop slowly over time and are categorised by numbers 1 to 4. Category 1 pressure sore symptoms include discoloured, warm, spongy or hard skin in the affected area. The area will not turn white when pressed and there may be pain/itchiness present. Category 2 pressure sores will show an open would or blister. Category 3 pressure sores are characterised by a deep wound that extends to deeper layers of the skin. When the pressure sore moves past the skin down to the muscle or bone it is a category 4 pressure sore.

Conventional Medical Treatment: Treatment dependent on severity and aims to aid to healing process and prevent infection. Minor sores can be relieved by changing position regularly and using specially designed mattresses and/or cushions. Alginate, hydrocolloid and antimicrobial dressings can be used to protect the sore and speed healing. Antibiotics will be prescribed if infection is present. Debridement, the removal of dead tissue via high-pressure water jets, ultrasound or scalpel, may be used to help the sore heal. Severe sores may require surgery to clean and seal the wound.

Prognosis: Prevention is better than cure. Pressure sores can be difficult to treat and heal. Without treatment, there is a serious risk of infection. Infection can lead to serious complications such as cellulitis, osteomyelitis and sepsis.

Holistic Advice: Change position regularly and check the skin every day for the early signs of pressure sores. Keep at risk areas of skin clean and moisturised. Stop smoking. Lose weight if required, eat a healthy balanced diet and drink plenty of fluids.

Prolapsed Intervertebral Disc

Definition: Protrusion of one of the shock-absorbing pads that lie between the vertebrae. Also known as a slipped disc.

Possible Causes: Intervertebral discs have a strong fibrous outer layer and a soft, gelatinous inner. A prolapsed disc occurs when the gel inside the core pushes outwards, distorting the shape of the disc. The outer coat can rupture, allowing the gel to leak out. The damaged disc can put pressure on an individual nerve or the whole spinal cord creating pain in any part of the body served by the affected nerve. Risk factors that may decrease the strength of the supporting connective tissue that holds the disc in place include age, awkward bending, heavy lifting, sitting for long periods, smoking, being overweight and having a back injury. Once weakened, the disc may slip.

General Signs and Symptoms: Most will experience pain, often beginning in the back and radiating to other parts of the body depending on which nerve is under pressure from the prolapsed disc. It can cause muscular weakness and spasm. The sciatic nerve is commonly affected, leading to sciatic pain that runs from the back of the pelvis, through the buttocks and down one or both legs, causing aching, numbness and tingling.

Conventional Medical Treatment: Given time the disc will often shrink back and so the pain ceases. Medication such as painkillers, non-steroidal anti-inflammatory drugs, corticosteroid injections and muscle relaxants may be prescribed to cope with the pain. In severe cases surgery may be recommended to remove the pressure on the nerve caused by the slipped disc.

Prognosis: For most, a combination of gentle exercise and painkillers will resolve the situation within about 4-6 weeks but it can be a serious problem and once there is a weakness, the condition may recur.

Holistic Advice: Regular exercise to keep the back strong and flexible, and ensuring that correct lifting techniques are used can help prevent this condition. Maintaining a good posture at all times, sleeping on a suitable mattress and not carrying any excess body weight also contribute to keeping the spine healthy and functional.

Prolapse (Uterine/Vaginal)

Definition: Uterine prolapse is where the uterus slips from its normal position and bulges into the vagina. Vaginal prolapse is where the top of the vagina sags down.

Possible Causes: Occurs when the muscle and tissue (known as the pelvic floor) that usually support the uterus and vagina weaken and cannot keep them place. The pelvic floor can weaken due to; pregnancy and childbirth, age and/or menopause, being overweight, long term constipation, having a hysterectomy and performing a job that requires excessive heavy lifting. Additionally, joint hypermobility syndrome, Marfan syndrome and Ehlers-Danlos syndromes can make prolapse more likely to occur.

General Signs and Symptoms: In some cases, there can be no symptoms. Generally, women will experience heaviness in the lower abdomen and vagina, discomfort or numbness during sexual intercourse, problems passing urine (increased need, leaking, and stress incontinence) and feeling or seeing a bulge/lump coming out of the vagina.

Conventional Medical Treatment: Recommended treatment will depend on the type of severity of the prolapse. If mild, lifestyle changes such as losing weight, avoiding heavy lifting and preventing/treating constipation may be advised. If severe pelvic floor exercises, hormone treatment, vaginal pessaries or surgery.

Prognosis: Not life threatening and mild symptoms can be relieved by non-invasive treatments combined with lifestyle changes. If surgery is required (severe cases), there can be complications such as infection, long-lasting pain, nerve damage, injury to surrounding organs and incontinence. Recovery from surgery should take around 4 – 6 weeks.

Holistic Advice: Maintain a healthy weight and eating a high fibre diet to avoid constipation. Stop smoking and avoid high impact exercise as well as heavy lifting.

Prostate Cancer

Definition: Cancer of the prostate.

Possible Causes: Exact causes are unknown but risk factors include age (more likely in over 50's), being of African-Caribbean or African descent, family history of prostate cancer and obesity.

General Signs and Symptoms: Develops very slowly so symptoms often only occur when the prostate is large enough to affect the urethra. This causes increased frequency of urination, needing to rush to the toilet, difficulty urinating, blood in the urine or semen and feeling like the bladder is not fully empty.

Conventional Medical Treatment: Initially the stage of the cancer will be determined to outline a treatment plan. In many cases, no treatment will be necessary, as the cancer will not affect the natural lifespan of the patient. Often the cancer will be monitored in order to delay treatment either through 'watchful waiting' or 'active surveillance'. A radical prostatectomy (surgery to remove the prostate) and radiotherapy can be performed on prostate cancer that has not spread beyond the prostate. To increase success of internal radiotherapy (brachytherapy), hormone treatment to reduce testosterone is often offered. For advanced prostate cancer which cannot be cured, treatment options include a combination of radiotherapy, hormone treatment and chemotherapy.

Prognosis: As prostate cancer often develops slowly, it is possible to live with it without treatment for a number of years. Surgery to remove the prostate will cause infertility, can have negative effects on the ability to get an erection, and can cause urinary incontinence. Radiotherapy can also have the same effect on the ability to get an erection and can also cause issues with the rectum/anus including diarrhoea, bleeding and discomfort. Brachytherapy has a higher risk of urinary issues than normal radiotherapy.

Holistic Advice: If you notice, any symptoms ensure you go and see your GP. Maintain a healthy weight. Practice pelvic floor exercise to strengthen the muscles to help with any urinary incontinence.

Prostatitis

Definition: Inflammation of the prostate gland. There are 3 main types – acute prostatitis, chronic bacterial prostatitis and chronic non-bacterial prostatitis.

Possible Causes: Acute prostatitis is uncommon and is caused by bacteria that enter the prostate from the urinary tract. Chronic prostatitis is also caused by bacterial infection of the prostate, but in this case the bacteria infection develops in the prostate and may then spread into the urinary tract. Chronic non bacterial prostatitis is the most common. Its cause is unknown but may be linked to problems in the immune system or nervous system, or from an undiscovered viral or bacterial infection.

General Signs and Symptoms: Acute prostatitis produces sudden and severe symptoms including a fever and severe pain in the pelvis, genitals, lower back, base of the penis and the buttocks. There may be a need to urinate frequently and urination, ejaculation and defaecation may be painful. Chronic prostatitis does not always show symptoms, but if symptoms do occur they tend to develop gradually and be mild but persistent, although they can fluctuate in severity from day to day. The symptoms for chronic prostatitis are the same as for acute prostatitis but some may also experience tiredness, joint and muscle pain.

Conventional Medical Treatment: Antibiotics can be used to treat cases of prostatitis caused by bacterial infection. Alpha blockers may also be used to relax the bladder muscles to help with urination. Laxatives can be used to help bowel movement. Non-bacterial prostatitis can be difficult to treat because of the lack of knowledge about its cause. Alpha blockers, paracetamol and ibuprofen are commonly prescribed to help treat the symptoms.

Prognosis: Most men make a full recovery but all types of prostatitis can recur.

Holistic Advice: Any prostate problem should be checked out to eliminate any sinister underlying cause.

Psoriasis

Definition: Inflammatory skin disorder.

Possible Causes: It is believed that the immune system may play a part by attacking healthy skin cells by mistake. There is an increased production of epidermal cells that results in immature cells reaching the surface of the skin. Psoriasis is often a family disease. It can be triggered by immune-depressing influences such as stress. Other triggers can include injury to skin, alcohol, smoking, some medicines and some immune disorders. Can be seasonal, in which case it is especially prevalent in spring and autumn.

General Signs and Symptoms: Raised, flaky, reddened, crusty areas covered with silvery scales, and chronic inflammation. Often appears on elbows, knees and scalp. The disease is divided into several varieties according to the shape and distribution of the patches.

Conventional Medical Treatment: Topical creams and ointments, phototherapy (exposing skin to certain types of ultraviolet light), oral and injected medication that reduces the production of skin cells.

Prognosis: Long-lasting (chronic) disease that can return at any time. There is no cure but the range of treatments can help alleviate symptoms. It is often cyclical, causing problems for a few weeks or month and then easing or stopping.

Holistic Advice: Stress must be treated. Anything that can help boost the immune system may help. Emollient creams can help to reduce scaliness. Eating raw vegetables and fresh fruit and drinking plenty of water can also be beneficial.

Psoriatic Arthritis

Definition: A form of arthritis that can affect some people with psoriasis.

Possible Causes: Linked to the skin condition psoriasis but it is unclear why some people develop psoriatic arthritis and some do not.

General Signs and Symptoms: Severity and areas affected can vary massively from person to person. Common symptoms include swelling, pain and stiffness in the joints particularly the knees, ankles, hands and feet. Flare-ups, where symptoms get noticeably worse, are hard to predict.

Conventional Medical Treatment: Treatment aims to reduce symptoms, improve quality of life and slow down/prevent permanent joint damage. Medication such as non-steroidal anti-inflammatory drugs, corticosteroids, anti-rheumatic drugs and biological therapies can all be trialled to find the most suitable for the individual.

Prognosis: There is no cure for psoriatic arthritis, but medication can help reduce the symptoms. If untreated it can get progressively worse and there is risk of permeant joint damage or deformity.

Holistic Advice: Practice self-care and aim to minimise stress. Eat a healthy balanced diet and take regular exercise.

Pulmonary Embolism

Definition: Obstruction of the blood flow to the lungs by one or more blood clots.

Possible Causes: A plug of material, called an embolus, gets lodged in a pulmonary artery, either partially or completely blocking the flow of blood. The word embolism refers to the blockage of an artery by the embolus. The embolus is usually made from pieces of a blood clot that have separated from a larger clot (thrombis) somewhere else in the body (often the legs) and travelled to the lungs in the bloodstream. Blood clots can be caused by slow blood flow, blood that clots too easily and blood vessel damage. Those with deep vein thrombosis (DVT) are at greater risk of pulmonary embolism. Other risk factors include inactivity, age, previous clots, family history, cancer and its treatments, combined contraceptive pill, hormone replacement therapy, pregnancy and obesity.

General Signs and Symptoms: Symptoms depend on the extent of the blockage. A large clot that prevents the flow of blood can cause sudden death. Single, very small clots may be asymptomatic. In most cases symptoms include shortness of breath, sharp chest pain, feeling faint and palpitations. The symptoms develop suddenly over a few minutes.

Conventional Medical Treatment: Treatment depends on the extent of the blockage. Anticoagulant drugs, such as heparin and warfarin, are usually given to help prevent existing clots from getting bigger and new clots from forming. Long term use of anticoagulants may be required. Emergency surgery may even be needed to remove the clot.

Prognosis: 1 in 3 massive pulmonary embolisms result in death. Those that survive the first few days are likely to make a full recovery. Those with recurrent minor pulmonary embolism may remain short of breath.

Holistic Advice: This is a medical emergency requiring urgent hospitalisation. The risk can be reduced by not smoking, losing any excess weight, taking regular exercise and eating a balanced healthy diet.

Pulmonary Fibrosis

Definition: The end result of a large number of conditions that cause a build-up of scar tissue in the lungs.

Possible Causes: Usually caused by inflammation, scarring or both from other lung conditions. The scarring and inflammation makes it difficult for oxygen to get to the blood. Most commonly caused by hypersensitivity pneumonitis, pneumoconiosis (lung diseases caused by workplace dust/particle inhalation), connective tissues diseases and autoimmune diseases. Some medications, antibiotics and cancer treatments such as chemotherapy can also cause pulmonary fibrosis. When there is no clear cause it is known as idiopathic pulmonary fibrosis (IPF). IPF has been linked to exposure to dust, viral infections, family history of IPF, smoking and gastro-oesophageal reflux disease though there is no conclusive evidence that any of these are a direct cause.

General Signs and Symptoms: Depending on the cause. Most commonly, the first symptom experienced is breathlessness upon exertion. This can progress to breathlessness at rest. Other signs include a persistent cough, fatigue and clubbing of the fingers.

Conventional Medical Treatment: Treatment will be dependent on cause, with an aim to slow the damage to the lungs. Any medication causing problems to the lungs should be ceased. If caused by hypersensitivity pneumonitis and pneumoconiosis it will be advised to completely avoid the particles/dust/fumes or environments that trigger symptoms. Steroids to reduce inflammation can also treat hypersensitivity pneumonitis. For IFP, medications can be used to slow the development of scarring in the lungs. Oxygen therapy can be used to treat breathlessness. In very few cases, a lung transplant may be recommended.

Prognosis: There is no currently no cure and long term prognosis is dependent on cause. Some will respond very well to treatment and some will rapidly deteriorate. Minor health problems, such as catching a cold, can cause complications.

Holistic Advice: Stop smoking. Exercise regularly and eat a healthy balanced diet. Try to keep away from anyone with a cold or chest infection. Practice good hand hygiene.

Pyelonephritis

Definition: Kidney infection resulting in the inflammation of one or both of the kidneys. Because the kidneys are a part of the urinary tract, pyelonephritis is classed as a urinary tract infection (UTI).

Possible Causes: Usually caused by a bacterial infection (typically e-coli bacteria that live in the colon) that gets transferred from the anus to the urethra and then moves up from the bladder to the kidney(s). Occasionally a kidney infection can develop from a bacterial or fungal skin infection, and bacteria may also be carried to the kidneys in the blood. Other risk factors include blockages of the urinary tract, kidney stones, conditions that prevent the bladder from fully emptying and a weakened immune system. People with diabetes mellitus are more likely to suffer from urinary tract infections because the presence of glucose in the urine may encourage bacterial growth. Pyelonephritis can also be caused if bacteria are introduced to the urinary tract during catheterization. Women, particularly those who are sexually active, are at greater risk.

General Signs and Symptoms: Typical symptoms include a fever, shivering, pain in the side of the abdomen, nausea, vomiting, diarrhoea and back pain. Symptoms usually develop quickly. If other parts of the urinary tract are affected symptoms associated with cystitis can also be experienced, e.g. cloudy or strong smelling urine, a feeling of incomplete emptying of the bladder, blood in the urine, and lower abdominal pain.

Conventional Medical Treatment: Antibiotics are used to tackle the infection. Any underlying cause may also be treated.

Prognosis: Most recover fully within about 2 weeks.

Holistic Advice: Drink plenty of fluids. Empty the bladder frequently and completely. After going to the toilet wipe from front to back, wash before and after sex, and urinate after sex.

Raynaud's

Definition: Sudden, intermittent narrowing of the arteries in the hands or, rarely, the feet.

Possible Causes: Muscular spasm of the artery walls restricts the blood supply to the fingers or toes. In most cases it is not caused by an underlying condition and is therefore called primary Raynaud's. Secondary Raynaud's is caused by an underlying condition, particularly scleroderma (thickening of the skin) and autoimmune conditions such as rheumatoid arthritis and lupus. Risk factors include exposure to the cold, side effect of some medications, exposure to vibration, smoking, stress, anxiety and injury or overuse of the fingers.

General Signs and Symptoms: Fingers or toes become pale and then blue and feel numb or tingly. The fingers or toes become very red as the blood returns to the tissues. It may cause a painful burning sensation. In primary Raynaud's all the fingers on both hands are usually affected at once. In secondary Raynaud's symptoms often begin only on a couple of fingers on one hand. Raynaud's is most common in women aged 15-45 and is usually mild.

Conventional Medical Treatment: Preventative measures such as keeping warm and not smoking may be sufficient to deal with mild symptoms. In severe cases medication can be given to dilate the small blood vessels, and a surgical procedure can be used to cut or strip out the nerves to the affected area to reduce the pain. As a last resort, intravenous infusion therapy can be used to introduce a drug into the body that dilates the small blood vessels and helps prevent blood clotting. For secondary Raynaud's, the underlying cause of the problem will be investigated and, if found, it will be treated accordingly.

Prognosis: Usually harmless but severe cases may lead to skin ulcers or gangrene on the tips of the digits affected.

Holistic Advice: Keep warm, avoid direct contact with cold objects, reduce caffeine intake and give up smoking.

Renal Colic

Definition: The pain associated with stones blocking a part or parts of the urinary tract including the kidneys, ureters, bladder and urethra.

Possible Causes: Stones are formed when minerals such as calcium and uric acid fuse in the urine to create hard crystals. Risk factors that increase the chance of stones forming are a diet high in protein, family history of stones, dehydration, obesity and urinary tract infections. Having other metabolic disorders such a hyperparathyroidism can increase the chance of forming stones.

General Signs and Symptoms: Smaller stones may not cause any symptoms. Larger stones can block the ureter (tube that takes urine from the kidney to the bladder). This blockage can cause intense pain in the ribs and lower abdomen, pain the lower back or groin and nausea/vomiting. This pain often occurs in waves lasting anywhere between 20 minutes to 1 hour. Additional symptoms of stones include painful urination, blood in the urine, change in urination habits and cloudy or foul smelling urine.

Conventional Medical Treatment: Small stones may pass through the body and out via the urine without much trouble. If a large stone has caused a blockage, extracorporeal shock wave lithotripsy (ESWL) might be used to break up the stone into smaller fragments. Alternatively, a ureteroscopy might be used to grab and remove the stone through the urethra. Painkillers and anti-inflammatories will be given to relieve the pain and swelling.

Prognosis: Relatively little harm if treated quickly. If not treated, urinary stones can lead to other conditions such as urinary tract infections or kidney damage.

Holistic Advice: Drink plenty of water. Limit the amount of salt, protein and fizzy drinks in the diet. Maintain a healthy weight.

Renal Failure

Definition: Where the kidneys no longer function. Can be acute (sudden) or chronic (long lasting, over time).

Possible Causes: Acute renal failure (ARF) happens when the kidneys suddenly stop filtering the blood and do not remove waste products. It is most likely to occur when blood flow to the kidney is disrupted (e.g. via injury), swelling in the kidney (from medication or infection), sudden blockage (kidney stone) or very high blood pressure. Chronic renal failure (CRF) develops slowly overtime, usually because of chronic kidney disease. Other causes include high blood pressure, uraemia, chronic glomerulonephritis, diabetes, polycystic kidney disease, kidney infection or problems with the urinary tract.

General Signs and Symptoms: Symptoms of ARF can include swelling of the hands/feet/face, high blood pressure, abnormal blood and urine tests, internal bleeding, confusion, seizures and in some instances coma. CRF symptoms develop slowly and may not show until kidney function reduces to 20% or less. Signs can include abnormal blood and urine tests, high blood pressure, unexplained weight loss, anaemia, nausea, vomiting, shortness of breath, chest pain, confusion, seizures, coma, jaundice, fatigue and swelling of the hands/feet/face.

Conventional Medical Treatment: For ARF, treating the underlying cause is the first step. This can include medication to treat high blood pressure, kidney stones or diabetes. For CRF treating high blood pressure and/or diabetes can slow the progression toward kidney failure. The most successful treatment for kidney failure is a kidney transplant. The kidney can come from a living or deceased donor. If a donor cannot be found or transplant is not suitable, dialysis can be given to artificially filter the blood.

Prognosis: ARF can be fatal but quick treatment can reverse the effects and restore normal or near normal function. CRF prognosis will depend on the co-morbidities and stage of failure. Dialysis does not cure kidney failure and will only serve to prolong life. Kidney transplant will cure kidney failure but there are additional risks from surgery and immune system reactions (rejection of the new kidney) to consider.

Holistic Advice: Eat a healthy diet and maintain a healthy weight. Limit foods high in salt and potassium. Avoid alcohol. Maintain good control over diabetes if you have it.

Repetitive Strain Injury (RSI)

Definition: Generalised term to describe pain in joints, muscles and tendons following overuse or repetitive movements. Also known as RSI.

Possible Causes: Overuse of the muscles and tendons. Repetitive activities (working on an assembly line, at a computer or at a supermarket checkout), poor posture, high-intensity activity with not enough rest and working in awkward positions can all cause repetitive strain injury. The use of vibrating equipment in the workplace can increase the risk of developing RSI.

General Signs and Symptoms: Can ranged from mild to severe and often develop over time. Most common in the upper body such as the forearm, elbows, wrists, hands, neck and shoulder. Initially symptoms occur when the repetitive action is being performed and can include pain, aching, stiffness, throbbing, tingling, numbness, weakness and cramp. Over time, these symptoms can become constant and swelling in the affected area may become apparent. Working in cold environments can exacerbate symptoms.

Conventional Medical Treatment: Dependent on symptoms and if there is an underlying condition present. RSI can often be treated at home with ice packs, rest and painkillers. Physiotherapy can be used for posture advice. Pain receptor blocking medications may be prescribed for severe symptoms. Specific medical conditions such as carpal tunnel syndrome or Dupuytren's contracture could require surgery to relieve symptoms.

Prognosis: Symptoms usually disappear when the repetitive activity is reduced or stopped.

Holistic Advice: Take regular breaks at work. Take regular exercise and maintain good posture.

Rheumatoid Arthritis

Definition: Chronic autoimmune disease that causes the joints to become painful, swollen, stiff and deformed.

Possible Causes: The immune system attacks the lining of the joints, causing swelling and inflammation. If the inflammation persists it may damage the ends of the bone and the cartilage that covers them. Tendons and ligaments may also become worn and deformity of the joint arises. The actual cause of this autoimmune condition is unknown. Some think it may be triggered by an infection or virus but nothing is proven. It is more common in women and so oestrogen may play a part. There is some evidence that it may run in families.

General Signs and Symptoms: The condition causes joint pain, stiffness and warmth and redness in the affected area. The joints may appear bumpy. Rheumatoid arthritis tends to develop slowly with the small joints, commonly the in the hands, being affected first. The condition has "flare-ups" and the symptoms tend to worsen with each one. The pain and stiffness is usually worse in the mornings. Other general symptoms such as tiredness, poor appetite and loss of weight may show and, because the condition can be painful and debilitating, depression is quite common.

Conventional Medical Treatment: There is no cure. The treatment focuses on controlling the symptoms and reducing further joint damage by slowing the progression of the disease. Many different drugs are available, some for the pain and some to slow the progression of the disease. Surgery can be used to correct joint deformities and reduce pain. Physiotherapy and, as the disease progresses, help with day-to-day life may be necessary.

Prognosis: Lifelong drug treatment may be needed to control the symptoms. Some will become severely disabled. Complications include carpal tunnel syndrome, ruptured tendons and bursitis, and the inflammation may affect other parts of the body including the lungs, heart, blood vessels and the eyes.

Holistic Advice: Take gentle, regular exercise and maintain a healthy diet. Support groups can offer advice and self-help guidance for the sufferer and his/her family.

Ringworm

Definition: A common superficial fungal skin infection. Also known as tinea corporis.

Possible Causes: Predominantly caused by the dermatophyte fungi trichophyton rubrum. Fungal spores are shed from infected skin and can be spread to other people by close contact and the sharing of bedding, towels, combs and clothing. Ringworm can also be caused by trichophyton interdigitale, trichophyton tonsurans and microsporum canis (from cats and dogs).

General Signs and Symptoms: Most commonly presents as a ring shaped red rash with a raised scaly edge. This rash can develop anywhere on the body and can grow, spread or multiply.

Conventional Medical Treatment: Topical antifungal creams are most commonly used to treat ringworm. Sprays or gels may also be recommended depending on where the rash location. Oral antifungal treatments may be used if topical antifungal treatments are ineffective.

Prognosis: Large majority of cases resolve after treatment. Recurrence is possible if treatment is stopped prematurely or if the source of infection is left untreated.

Holistic Advice: Keep skin clean and dry. Wear loose fitting clothing. Do not scratch or pick at the rash. Avoid close contact and sharing bedding, towels, combs or clothing with infected persons.

Rosacea

Definition: A chronic skin condition that mainly affects the face. Formerly known as acne rosacea.

Possible Causes: Exact cause is unknown but it is thought that there could be links to inflammatory responses in the skin caused by the immune system. There are triggers that can exacerbate symptoms including sun exposure, hot weather, stress, alcohol, spicy foods and strenuous exercise. Rosacea typically begins after the age of 30, is more common in women and people with lighter skin who blush or flush easily. This is a possibility that this condition runs in families.

General Signs and Symptoms: Rosacea is initially characterised by redness or blushing across the nose, cheeks, forehead and chin. This redness may come and go and can be accompanied by sensitivity to water or skincare products on the skin. As the condition progresses the redness can become more persistent and blood vessels will become more visible. Severe rosacea can cause bumps/pimples (without a yellow or black head), thickening or swollen skin across the nose and irritated eyes. Men appear to suffer with more severe symptoms than women do.

Conventional Medical Treatment: Topical creams can be used to control redness and reduce bumps/pimples. Long term oral antibiotics may also be prescribed. IPL (intense pulsed light) treatment can be used to remove visible blood vessels. Referral to a dermatologist may be appropriate.

Prognosis: There is no cure but symptoms can be managed with consistent treatments and avoidance of triggers that cause flushing. If not treated the condition can get worse.

Holistic Advice: Where possible, avoid possible triggers that cause flushing. Protect the skin from the sun using high factor sun cream. Do not use any skincare products that cause burning, irritation or additional redness.

<u>Sarcoidosis</u>

Definition: A rare autoimmune condition that causes granulomas (patches of red and swollen tissue) to develop, particularly in the lungs and on the skin.

Possible Causes: Believed to be caused by the immune system overreacting and attacking the body's own tissues, causing inflammation. It is not known why the immune system does this. Can occur in more than one family member but there is no evidence to suggest it is genetic. Sarcoidosis is more common in women and usually occurs in adults between the ages of 20 and 40.

General Signs and Symptoms: Dependent on which organ is affected. Pulmonary sarcoidosis (lungs) causes shortness of breath and a persistent dry cough. In small cases, pain can be felt in the chest. On the skin, tender red bumps/patches develop as well as rashes. These are usually found on the shins but can be anywhere. If other organs are affected swollen glands, tiredness, painful joints, sore eyes, heart rhythm issues, blocked nose, kidney stones and headache can all be experienced.

Conventional Medical Treatment: Treatment is not always necessary and symptoms may gradually subside over a period of months or years. Paracetamol and ibuprofen can be used to treat any pain or flare ups. If treatment is required steroid tablets are usually prescribed to relieve symptoms and reduce damage to the affected organs. If steroids are not enough to control symptoms, immunosuppressant medication can be used.

Prognosis: Symptoms fluctuate over time and can usually be managed at home. Most will see their symptoms disappear over a few months or years. In some cases, the condition can gradually worsen causing permanent organ damage.

Holistic Advice: Stop smoking and avoid exposure to dust/chemicals/fumes and toxic gases. Eat a healthy balanced diet and exercise regularly. Drink plenty of fluids.

Scabies

Definition: An very infectious and itchy skin rash. Also known as sarcoptic itch.

Possible Causes: Caused when a parasitic mite called sarcoptes scabiei var. hominis burrows into the surface of the skin. Scabies is most commonly transmitted via skin-to-skin contact with an infected person. Less commonly caught from bedding or towels that have been used by an infected person.

General Signs and Symptoms: Characterised by a very itchy rash which often begins in between the fingers but can appear anywhere on the body. Over time, the rash may spread across the body (except the head) and turn into small spots which can appear red on lighter skin tones. There may be visible tracks where the mites have burrowed under the skin. The rash may occur on the head a neck in children or people with weakened immune systems.

Conventional Medical Treatment: Topical insecticides applied to the whole body to eradicate the mites and their eggs. Treatment should be repeated 1 week after initial application. Every person in the household should be treated regardless of presence of symptoms. Antibiotics may be prescribed for any secondary infections.

Prognosis: Generally not considered a serious condition and most cases should resolve after treatment. The itch may persist for weeks post treatment. Scabies can make pre-existing skin conditions like eczema and psoriasis worse. Left untreated crusted scabies, where the skin is infected with thousands/millions of mites, can occur. Secondary infections can occur due to scratching and include impetigo, cellulitis and sepsis.

Holistic Advice: Do not have close contact or share bedding/clothing/towels with other people until treatment is complete. Do not scratch the rash. Wash all bedding and clothing on the first day of treatment and place any clothing that cannot be washed in a sealed bag for at least 3 days.

Scars

Definition: A patch or line of tissue that remains after a wound has healed. Can be internal and external.

Possible Causes: Natural part of healing process that occurs after body tissue has been damaged, in which the body produces more of the protein collagen. Abnormal scars can develop if the wound becomes infected, when there is a loss of a large patch of skin, and after serious burns. Thick, lumpy and raised scars are called keloid scars and often become bigger than the original wound. The exact cause is unknown but it is thought to be due to an overproduction collagen during the healing process. Keloid scars often run in families but can affect anyone. They can occur after very minor skin damage and sometimes form months or years after the initial injury.

General Signs and Symptoms: External scars are visible. Scarring can be worse on more mobile areas of the body that continue to move during the healing process. Scars gradually become smoother and softer. Abnormal scars such as keloid scars can be itchy, painful and unsightly. Keloid scars are usually shiny, hairless, thick and rubbery.

Conventional Medical Treatment: Drugs may be prescribed to help break down scar tissue. Laser treatment and surgery can be used on severe cases to improve the appearance.

Prognosis: The affect a scar has on the person's life is largely dependent on how they feel about it. Scars tend to fade with time but can have detrimental psychological effects. If a person has had one keloid scar they have an increased chance of developing them again.

Holistic Advice: Creams or supplements containing vitamin E can speed up the healing process. Eggs and leafy green vegetables are rich in vitamin E. Make-up can be used to camouflage scars. How the person feels about themselves and the impact the scar has on their life should be addressed. The severity of the scarring can be minimized at the time of the injury by keeping the wound clean. Don't pick scabs or spots!

Sciatica

Definition: Pain originating from the sciatic nerve.

Possible Causes: Sciatica results from the compression or damage to the sciatic nerve or its roots. This can be brought on by a slipped disc, narrowing of the spinal cord, degeneration of the intervertebral discs, osteoarthritis, muscle spasm, injury and additional pressure on the spine during pregnancy, but sometimes the cause is unknown.

General Signs and Symptoms: Pain in the lower back and buttock that travels down the back of the thigh and outside of the leg, often going into the outside of the foot. May cause numbness, muscle weakness or tingling in the legs and feet. Movement usually makes the pain worse.

Conventional Medical Treatment: Acute (short-term) sciatica can usually be managed with a combination of painkillers, anti-inflammatory drugs, exercise and hot/cold packs. In more severe cases stronger painkillers may be necessary and physiotherapy or chiropractic may be required. Surgery can be used to reduce the pressure on the sciatic nerve by removing discs, fusing vertebrae, or by widening the spinal cord.

Prognosis: Mild sciatica does not usually last longer than 6 weeks and tends to sort itself out without treatment. Sciatica can recur unless the underlying cause is rectified.

Holistic Advice: Look into general posture and the work/home environment e.g. height of chairs, desks and computer screen. The shortening of the piriformis muscle can often cause sciatic pain, so soft tissue manipulation (including muscle energy techniques) can also be beneficial. Bed rest may provide temporary relief but can make the symptoms worse. Walking and gentle stretching is of benefit. Acupuncture may help relieve the pain. Some find regular "maintenance" visits to an osteopath or chiropractor beneficial.

Scleroderma

Definition: A rare autoimmune disorder that causes connective tissue to harden and thicken. There are two major types, localised scleroderma (affecting the skin) and systemic sclerosis (affecting the skin, internal organs and blood circulation).

Possible Causes: Exact cause is unknown. It is thought that there could be links to the immune system causing an over production of collagen in the connective tissue. Having a close family member with the condition may increase the risk of developing scleroderma.

General Signs and Symptoms: Localised scleroderma is the mildest form and there are two types known as morphoea and linear. Morphoea can occur anywhere on the body and is characterised by itchy, discoloured oval patches. Linear occurs in lines along the face, scalp, legs or arms and can sometimes affect the underlying muscle or bone. Systemic sclerosis also has two types, limited cutaneous and diffuse. Limited cutaneous is milder and often starts as Raynaud's, affecting the skin on the face, lower arms, lower legs and feet. Alongside the thickening of the skin there may be red spots and hard lumps under the skin. It can progress to the lungs and digestive system causing heartburn and problems swallowing (dysphagia). Symptoms often get worse over time. Diffuse is more likely to affect skin all over the body and internal organs. Additional symptoms include weight loss, fatigue and joint pain. Further issues depend on what internal organs are affected. Symptoms come on suddenly and get worse over the initial couple of years before plateauing.

Conventional Medical Treatment: Treatment aims to relieve symptoms and attempt to stop the condition getting worse. Medication can be used to reduce the activity of the immune system, improve circulation and control pain. Steroids can be prescribed to help with muscle and joint pain. In severe cases, surgery can be used to remove hard lumps under the skin or loosen tight muscles.

Prognosis: There is currently no cure for scleroderma but symptoms can be managed with treatment.

Holistic Advice: Moisturise the affected areas to keep the skin supple and reduce itchiness. Eat a healthy balanced diet, exercise regularly and stop smoking.

Seasonal Affective Disorder

Definition: A type of depression that has a seasonal pattern. Often abbreviated to SAD.

Possible Causes: Thought to be linked to the reduced exposure to sunlight in the winter months. The lack of light may affect the hormones melatonin (influencing sleep patterns) and serotonin (affecting mood, appetite and sleep). Reduced sunlight may also affect the body's natural internal clock. Risk factors include family history of depression, adverse childhood experiences, and psychological and social factors.

General Signs and Symptoms: Depression is more apparent in the winter months, resulting in being less active, putting on weight and sleeping more. Sufferers may feel tired, stressed, anxious and generally unhappy. The usual symptoms of depression are commonly present, e.g. low self esteem, tearfulness and feelings of despair.

Conventional Medical Treatment: Antidepressants used for other forms of depression may help. Cognitive behavioural therapy (CBT) can help create an individualised programme to help gradually change the way people think/feel about situations and how to cope with them. Talking therapies such as counselling and psychodynamic psychotherapy can also be used. Light therapy, to expose the body to more light during the winter months, may give short-term relief. This involves wearing a light visor or sitting in front of a light box.

Prognosis: Like any form of depression, it can be difficult to live with. Treatments can offer relief. Symptoms usually relieve when Spring arrives.

Holistic Advice: Try to get as much natural sunlight as possible throughout the day. Make living and working environments light and bright using full spectrum light bulbs or natural light. Take regular exercise, preferably outdoors, and eat a healthy, well balanced diet. Avoid stressful situations and talk to family and friends about feelings and concerns.

Sebaceous Cysts

Definition: A sebaceous cyst is a harmless swelling under the skin that may become infected. The term "cyst" is a general term used to describe an enclosed sac that may contain air, fluids or semi-solid material, but not normally pus. Cysts can appear in various locations of the body, e.g. ovarian cysts, epididymal cysts and breast cysts. Cysts are usually harmless but depending on their location can be malignant. We will focus on sebaceous cysts here.

Possible Causes: Commonly caused by the inflammation of a hair follicle (also called follicular cyst). The sac of the cyst fills with a fatty, white, semi-solid material made up of dead skin cells and sebum.

General Signs and Symptoms: A smooth, usually painless lump under the skin. Some cysts have a dark central pore. They commonly occur on the scalp, face, trunk and genitals but may appear anywhere. They may grow large and become unsightly. If a cyst gets infected by bacteria it can become inflamed and painful and may eventually burst.

Conventional Medical Treatment: Can be left untreated if the cyst is not causing problems. Should a cyst become infected, it can be treated with antibiotics or can be incised and drained. Problematic cysts can be surgically removed under local anaesthetic. If not completely removed they may return.

Prognosis: No serious health implications.

Holistic Advice: Boost the immune system. Maintain good skin hygiene.

Sepsis

Definition: A life-threatening condition that occurs when the immune system overreacts to infection and begins damaging the body's own tissues. Also referred to as septicaemia or blood poisoning.

Possible Causes: Any infection can lead to sepsis. Those particularly at risk are babies under 1, people over 75, people undergoing chemotherapy, people who had recently had surgery or serious illness and people with diabetes. Women who have recently given birth, had a miscarriage or abortion are also at risk. Sepsis cannot be caught or spread.

General Signs and Symptoms: Sepsis signs can be vague and very difficult to spot as there are many possible symptoms that are similar to other conditions. In older children and adults, symptoms include confusion, slurred speech, blue/pale/blotchy skin, a rash that does not fade when a glass is rolled over it and difficulty breathing (including breathlessness and rapid breathing). In babies and young children symptoms include, blue/pale/blotchy skin, a rash that does not fade when a glass is rolled over it, difficulty breathing, not responding as normal, disinterested in normal activities, weak/high pitched cry and being sleepier than normal.

Conventional Medical Treatment: Urgent medical treatment at hospital is required in all cases. Antibiotics to treat the infection will be prescribed and administered. Depending on the symptoms, treatment in intensive care and surgery to remove the infection are a possibility.

Prognosis: Most people make a full recovery although this can take some time. If not treated early, sepsis can progress to septic shock which will cause the organs to fail. Long-term effects are sometimes referred to as post-sepsis syndrome, which can last months or even years. Symptoms of this include lethargy, difficulty sleeping, lack of appetite, frequent illness, anxiety, depression, nightmares and post-traumatic stress disorder (PTSD).

Holistic Advice: Take steps to prevent infection such as practice good hand hygiene, clean for wounds properly and ensure the full course of prescribed antibiotics are taken. Pregnant women, older people and babies should ensure a complete and up to date vaccination record.

Severe Acute Respiratory Syndrome (SARS)

Definition: A coronavirus known as SARS CoV which is believed to have mutated from a coronavirus found in small mammals allowing it to spread to humans.

Possible Causes: A mutated strain of coronavirus that is thought to have spread from small mammals to humans in 2002. It is highly contagious and spread by small droplets from the cough or sneeze of an infected person, similarly to the common cold or flu. If someone breathes in these droplets, they can become infected (direct transmission). Infection can also be spread indirectly via handling objects that an infected person has touched with unwashed hands. People over the age of 65 are at particular risk of severe complications.

General Signs and Symptoms: Initial flu like symptoms begin 2 – 7 days after infection. First symptoms include fever, fatigue, headaches, chills, muscle pain, loss of appetite and diarrhoea. The infection then moves to the lungs causing additional symptoms such as dry cough and breathing issues. In severe cases, the levels of oxygen in the blood can be significantly reduced.

Conventional Medical Treatment: There is currently no cure for SARS. Suspected SARS cases should be admitted to hospital immediately and kept in isolation. Treatment is supportive and can include assisted breathing (via a ventilator), antibiotics (to treat pneumonia), antiviral medicine and high doses of steroids to reduce inflammation.

Prognosis: During the initial outbreak approximately 1 in 10 people who contracted SARS died. Over half of the total deaths were in the over 65 age group. Lack of proven effectiveness of treatment methods is still a concern.

Holistic Advice: Practice good hand and respiratory hygiene.

Shin Splints

Definition: Pain along the shin bone (tibia). Also known as medial tibial stress syndrome.

Possible Causes: Most commonly caused by impact exercise such as running. There is a higher chance of developing shin splints if the person has poor running technique or has quickly increased the amount of exercise they do after being inactive for a long period of time.

General Signs and Symptoms: Pain and tenderness along the front of the lower leg. Running or jumping on hard surfaces can exacerbate symptoms.

Conventional Medical Treatment: Symptoms often get better with treatment at home. Rest and taking painkillers will usually help. Using ice packs and switching to exercise with less impact such as yoga or swimming can aid recovery.

Prognosis: Symptoms usually pass in a couple of weeks.

Holistic Advice: Warm up before exercise. Gradually increase distance and intensity of exercise over time and do not rush back to the exercise level that caused the shin splints. Ensure that footwear is in good condition and provides support.

Shingles

Definition: An infection of a nerve and the area of skin that follows its path. Also known as Herpes zoster.

Possible Causes: Caused by the herpes varicella-zoster virus. This virus also causes chickenpox and can remain dormant in nerve cells until triggered later in life. It is thought that stress or ill health may cause the reactivation of the virus. It most commonly occurs in those aged 50-70, and those with a reduced immunity are at greatest risk. The herpes varicella-zoster virus is contagious and, although it will not cause shingles in another, direct contact with open blisters, which typify shingles, may cause chicken pox in a person who is not immune to this disease.

General Signs and Symptoms: The early symptoms of tingling and localised pain are followed by a painful rash of blisters that erupt along a path of a nerve, typically only on one side of the body. It usually affects the skin on the chest, abdomen or face. Other symptoms may include a fever, myalgia and tiredness. The blisters form scabs within 3-4 days and drop off several days later, possibly leaving scars. Discomfort may continue long after the rash has disappeared. This pain is called postherpetic neuralgia.

Conventional Medical Treatment: Antiviral drugs may be prescribed and painkillers may be used to reduce the discomfort. Calamine lotion may help the rash, as may wearing loose fitting clothing and keeping the rash as clean as possible to avoid bacterial infection. Antihistamines may help to relieve the itching. Anticonvulsant drugs may be prescribed to ease any postherpetic neuralgia.

Prognosis: There is no cure but most recover within 4-6 weeks, although postherpetic neuralgia may last several months. The treatments can only help ease the symptoms. The infection may recur.

Holistic Advice: Try to maintain healthy immune system and reduce stress levels. Try to prevent spreading the virus by not sharing towels, playing contact sports or swimming.

Sickle Cells Anaemia

Definition: An inherited disease that affects the shape of the red blood cells. The most serious of a group of disorders known as sickle cell disease.

Possible Causes: Sickle cell anaemia is inherited genetically. The parents may not have sickle cell themselves and only carry the gene that causes it. It is more common in people of African or Caribbean descent.

General Signs and Symptoms: Symptoms can be wide ranging but most commonly are painful episodes (sickle cell crises), regular infections and anaemia (low red blood cell count). Sickle cell crises can be severely painful and occur when blood vessels in the body become blocked. Often affecting one part of the body (hands/feet, ribs, spine, pelvis, abdomen) crises last up to 7 days on average. Cold weather, dehydration, stress and strenuous exercise can trigger crises. Other symptoms include delayed growth, gallstones, bone/joint pain, leg ulcers, strokes, eyesight issues, high blood pressure and kidney issues.

Conventional Medical Treatment: Some sickle cell crises can be managed at home using painkillers, drinking water, heat pads and distraction techniques to take the mind off the pain. For frequent painful crises, medication called can be taken to reduce the 'stickiness' of the red blood cells. Severe crises may require hospital treatment where painkillers such as morphine will be prescribed. To prevent infection, some people will need to take daily antibiotics.

Prognosis: Usually requires lifelong management and treatment. Extra precautions should be taken when going under general anaesthetic.

Holistic Advice: Take steps to try to reduce the incidence of crises by drinking plenty of fluids, avoiding extreme temperatures and avoiding very strenuous exercise. Learn and practice relaxation techniques such as breathing exercises. Avoid alcohol and smoking. Reduce the risk of infection by practicing good food and hand hygiene.

Sinusitis

Definition: Inflammation of the lining of the sinuses.

Possible Causes: Commonly caused by a viral infection (e.g. common cold or flu) but can be bacterial. The resulting inflammation causes the sinuses to block which results in mucus collecting in them, which may then create a secondary bacterial infection. Sinusitis can also be triggered or worsened by irritants (e.g. smoke and air pollution), allergic conditions (e.g. hay fever and asthma) and anything that narrows the nasal passages (e.g. nasal polyps and structural defects). Sufferers of cystic fibrosis (which causes a build up of mucus in the body) are more likely to develop sinusitis. Those with reduced immunity are more susceptible to the infections that cause sinusitis.

General Signs and Symptoms: Facial pain, chronic dull ache around the cheekbones, blocked or runny nose, discoloured nasal discharge, headache (especially when the head tips forward), and a raised temperature. The sufferer may also feel tired and unwell and may experience a loss of taste and smell and develop a cough and bad breath.

Conventional Medical Treatment: Painkillers and decongestants can be used to relieve the facial pain and help the blocked nose. If symptoms persist, antibiotics may be given if there is a bacterial infection and steroid sprays or drops can help reduce the inflammation. Surgery can be performed to widen and improve the function of the sinuses.

Prognosis: Often clears up by itself within about two and a half weeks.

Holistic Advice: Avoid dairy and wheat products as they may provoke excessive formation of mucus. Consider regular massage to boost the immune system. Facial massage, concentrating on the sinus points, can help to clear the congestion. Acupuncture may be beneficial. Steam inhalation may help to release the mucus. Drink plenty of water, exercise regularly and do not smoke.

Skin – Additional Characteristics and Conditions

General Information:

Areas of the skin may change colour or texture. This is may be due to ageing, injury, infection, environmental factors, lifestyle or an underlying disease. Some drugs may also affect the skin.

Minor blemishes and abnormalities are not always associated with underlying disorders and are unlikely to need treatment. However, if the colour or general condition of the skin changes when no obvious damage has occurred a Doctor should be consulted.

On the next page the following will be summarised:

- Broken Capillaries
- Comedones
- Crow's Feet
- Dehydrated Skin
- Dermatosis Papulosa Nigra
- Ephelides (Freckles)
- Lentigo
- Melia
- Naevus (Mole)
- Sensitive Skin
- Striae (Stretch Marks)
- Papilloma
- Port-wine Stain
- Thin Skin

Skin – Additional Characteristics and Conditions

Broken Capillaries: Small viable red blood vessels also known as telangiectases. Generally harmless with treatment sought to reduce appearance. Commonly seen in liver disease, Cushing syndrome or other skin conditions such as rosacea. Can also occur due to injury and the use of topical steroid medication.

Comedones: A clogged hair follicle (pore) in the skin. Can be open (blackhead) or closed (whitehead). Comedones are very common in acne but can occur without acne.

Crow's Feet: Wrinkles or fine lines occurring at the outside corner of the eye. A natural part of ageing and not linked to any underlying conditions.

Dermatosis Papulosa Nigra: Multiple small, smooth, dark brown or black papules on the face and neck. Most commonly seen in women with darker skin types. The usually develops in adolescence, the exact cause is unknown but there is thought to be a genetic link. They are usually left alone and any treatment would be for cosmetic purposes.

Dry/Dehydrated Skin: Skin that is lacking moisture in the outer layer (stratum corneum) which can result in cracks in the skins surface. Dry skin can affect anyone at any age but is commonly seen in older individuals (60 or above). Conditions such as hypothyroidism, chronic renal disease and malnutrition can cause dry skin. Frequent exposure to dry environments may also cause dry skin.

Ephelides: Commonly known as freckles, ephelides are an inherited characteristic and present as small light brown or tan marks on the skin. They are particularly common in fair skinned individuals and are not present at birth. Freckles increase in number following exposure to the sun, increasing in prominence in the summer and fading in the winter.

Lentigo: A flat or slightly raised pigmented area of skin with a clearly defined edge that does not fade in the winter months (unlike freckles). Common forms are due to UV radiation (sun damage, sunbeds and phototherapy) but can also be caused by radiation therapy. They are usually left alone but can be permanently removed by cryotherapy, intense pulsed light or pigment lasers.

Loss of Skin Sensation: Losing the sensation of temperature, touch or pain occurs when damage has been done to the peripheral nerves. Diabetic neuropathy is a common cause of loss of skin sensation.

Melia: Small harmless cysts containing keratin found just under the surface of the skin. Most commonly found on the face, melia present as small pearly-white bumps and rarely require treatment. Can occur due to other skin conditions such as lichen planus or at the site of an injury while the skin heals.

Naevus: Commonly known as a mole, naevus are common benign (non-cancerous) pigmented areas on the skin. They can be present at birth or acquired and can vary widely size and colour. The exact cause for developing moles is unknown however the number present is thought to depend on genetics, sun exposure and immune status. Having a greater number of moles on the body increases the risk of developing skin cancer (melanoma). Most moles are harmless and can be left alone but may be removed to exclude cancer or for cosmetic reasons.

Sensitive Skin: A lay term to describe skin with a reduced tolerance to the application of cosmetics or personal care products. Usually used to describe the face, sensitive skin often presents as stinging, itching, burning, redness, dryness, peeling or bumps. Can be caused by irritant contact dermatitis, allergic contact dermatitis, rosacea, dry skin and eczema.

Striae/Stretch Marks: Lines on the body that occur due to the tissue under the skin tearing. They tend to occur in areas where the skin undergoes progressive stretching but can be features of conditions such as Cushing and Marfan syndromes. Pregnant women, adolescents, body builders and overweight/obese people are susceptible. Stretch marks are very common and very rarely cause complications.

Papilloma: Generic term for an outward growing benign (non-cancerous) tumour on the skin. Skin tags and warts are common examples where the term papilloma may be used.

Port-wine Stain (Naevus flammus): A capillary vascular malformation present at birth. Characterised by a large flat patch of purple or dark red skin. The face is most commonly affected but it can occur anywhere on the body. Most remain unchanged over time but there is a small chance it will fade.

Thin Skin: Skin that tears, bruises or breaks easily is very common on the face, arms and hands of older adults due to a reduction in the production of collagen. Veins, tendons and bones may be visible through the skin. It is most commonly associated with ageing but can be caused by UV exposure, medication and lifestyle factors such as smoking.

Skin Cancer (Melanoma)

Definition: A type of skin cancer that begins in cells called melanocytes.

Possible Causes: Most commonly caused by too much exposure to UV radiation from the sun or tanning beds. The risk of developing melanoma increases with age and can also be affected by the number of moles a person has and the presence of birthmarks on the skin. People who have fair skin and those who sunburn easily are at a higher risk of melanoma. Conditions such as diabetes, Crohn's disease, ulcerative colitis and those with weakened immune systems are at greater risk.

General Signs and Symptoms: The most common sign is an unusual change to a mole, freckle or patch of skin. Normal moles are small, symmetrical, have smooth borders, even colour and do not change in appearance. The ABCDE checklist is used to highlight potential changes to the skin which could indicate melanoma.

- A – asymmetrical, refers to the shape of a mole. In melanoma, moles are likely to have uneven shapes.
- B – border, refers to the edge of the mole. In melanoma, moles are likely to have blurred or jagged borders.
- C – colour, refers to the colour of the mole. In melanoma, moles are likely to contain more than one shade.
- D – diameter, refers to the size of the mole. Melanomas are most commonly more than 6mm wide.
- E – evolving, refers to the mole changing in appearance. Melanomas may change size, shape and colour or become crusty and itchy.

Melanoma most commonly occurs on the back for men and on the legs for women. In very rare cases melanoma can begin in the eye, sometimes presenting a dark spot on the iris (coloured part of the eye) or affecting eyesight.

Conventional Medical Treatment: Dependent on the stage and the general health of the person. The most common treatment for melanoma that has not spread is surgery. In most lower stage cancers the melanoma and a small area of healthy tissue will be surgically removed. This is known as surgical excision and is done in combination with a skin graft or skin flap. If the cancer has spread to the lymph nodes further surgery will be required to remove the affected nodes. Targeted treatment and immunotherapies are used to slow disease progression in advanced melanoma where the cancer has spread to other part of the body. This could be combination with chemotherapy and radiotherapy.

Prognosis: If diagnosed early treatment is often successful. There is always a chance that melanoma can return, particularly if the cancer was widespread or advanced.

Holistic Advice: Prevention is better than cure! Avoid getting sunburnt and using sunbeds. Protect the skin using a high factor SPF or using clothing.

Skin Cancer (Non-Melanoma)

Definition: An umbrella term for a number of skin cancers that develop in the upper layers of the skin (epidermis), including basal cell carcinoma (BCC) and squamous cell carcinoma (SCC).

Possible Causes: Most commonly caused by too much exposure to UV radiation from the sun or tanning beds. The risk of developing non-melanoma increases with age. People who have fair skin and those who sunburn easily are at a higher risk of non-melanoma. Skin conditions such as solar keratosis and xeroderma pigmentosum increase the risk of non-melanoma as well as treatments for psoriasis and eczema. Conditions such as diabetes, Crohn's disease, ulcerative colitis and those with weakened immune systems are at greater risk. This is also true for conditions associated with the human papilloma virus (HPV) such as cervical cancer, genital warts and epidermodysplasia verruciformis.

General Signs and Symptoms: BCC does not usually spread to other parts of the body and commonly presents as a small, pearly white or pink lump or a red scaly patch which may or not have dark pigment within it. Over time the lump will increase in size and can become crusty, bleed or develop into an ulcer. SCC appears as a firm pink lump with a rough surface which can sometimes have a spiky horn like projection sticking up from the surface. It can be tender to touch, bleed easily and can develop into an ulcer. There is a very small chance that SCC will spread to the lymph nodes.

Conventional Medical Treatment: Dependent on type, location and if the cancer has spread. The main treatment for non-melanoma skin cancers is surgery. Surgical excision is used to remove the affected area along with a small section of healthy tissue to ensure the cancer is fully removed. It is often done in combination with a skin graft or skin flap. Very small cancers may be treated with curettage or cryotherapy. Photodynamic therapy, where the skin is treated with cream and strong light to kill the cancer, can be effective in BCC. Early BCC can also be treated with anti-cancer creams which encourage the immune system to attack the cancer. If surgery is not appropriate, BCC and SCC can be treated with radiotherapy and chemotherapy.

Prognosis: Treatment is often very successful. Surgery and photodynamic therapy can leave scarring. People who are immunocompromised have a slightly higher risk of the cancer returning.

Holistic Advice: Prevention is better than cure! Avoid getting sunburnt and using sunbeds. Protect the skin using a high factor SPF or using clothing.

Snoring

Definition: Noisy breathing during sleep.

Possible Causes: The noise associated with snoring is created when the soft tissues at the back of the nose, mouth and throat vibrate as the person breathes. This may be caused by an obstruction or narrowing of the pharynx leading from the back of the nasal cavity to the throat. This may be worsened by being overweight and more likely if lying on the back. Another possible cause is the relaxation or swelling of the tissue of the soft palette. Relaxation can be caused by alcohol or sedatives, and swelling can be caused by a throat infection or irritation of the palette by tobacco smoke. The vibration caused by the snoring itself further narrows the airway. The narrowing of the airways is called upper airway resistance syndrome (UARS). Severe snoring may be related to obstructive sleep apnea (OSA), where the airways may block for several seconds. The oxygen level falls, causing the person to come out of the deep sleep in order for normal breathing to resume.

General Signs and Symptoms: Snoring is characterised by snorting or rattling noises when asleep. In mild cases the snoring does no harm but in some cases breathing difficulties are experienced. UARS and OSA may have a detrimental affect on health, causing heart disease and strokes. Snoring can interrupt sleep patterns, causing tiredness, reducing concentration levels and increasing the risk of accidents.

Conventional Medical Treatment: Treatment is only usually required if snoring is affecting day to day life. Lifestyle changes such as reducing alcohol intake, losing weight and not smoking is usually the first requirement. If lifestyles changes do not help, devices are available to fit inside the mouth or nose to help keep the airways open. There are several surgical techniques that can be used as a last resort.

Prognosis: It may be possible to reduce snoring but a complete cure may not be possible.

Holistic Advice: Make the lifestyles changes as indicated above. Try not to roll over onto the back – sewing a golf ball to the back of nightwear can help this! Don't ignore emotional wellbeing.

Spasticity

Definition: Unusual tightness or stiffness in the muscles.

Possible Causes: Most commonly caused by damage or disruption to areas of the brain and spinal cord that control muscle and stretch reflexes. Conditions such as stroke, cerebral palsy and multiple sclerosis may display varying degrees of spasticity. Brain injury and spinal cord injury can also cause spasticity. Spasticity can be aggravated by sudden movements, infection, fatigue, stress, menstruation and pain.

General Signs and Symptoms: Severity and areas affected can vary widely from person to person but spasticity is most common in the legs. Muscle stiffness, muscle deformity, muscle fatigue and inhibition of muscle growth can be experienced. Movement is less precise and painful muscle spasms can occur. Pain, tightness and deformity of the joints is also common

Conventional Medical Treatment: Dependent on severity. Mild to moderate spasticity is often treated with gentle stretching and exercise. Spasticity that affects multiple muscles groups can be treated with various nerve blocking medications. More localised spasticity can be relieved with injections directly into the muscle.

Prognosis: Treatment can improve symptoms and provide a better quality of life. Untreated, spasticity can lead to frozen/immobilised joints and pressure sores.

Holistic Advice: Take regular gentle exercise and follow a gentle stretching programme.

Spina Bifida

Definition: A birth defect where the spine and spinal cord do not develop properly in the womb, causing a gap in the spine.

Possible Causes: A neural tube defect of which the exact cause is unknown. A significant risk factor is thought to be a lack of folic acid (vitamin B9) before and in the early stages of pregnancy. Some epilepsy and bipolar disorder medications can also increase the risk and should be avoided when trying to become pregnant. Family history of neural tube defects increase the risk of having a baby with spina bifida. Women who are obese and/or have diabetes have increased risk of having a child with spina bifida.

General Signs and Symptoms: Wide ranging symptoms dependent on the location of the gap in the spine. A gap higher in the spine is more likely to cause mobility issues and paralysis of the legs whereas a gap lower in the spine are more likely to cause continence issues (both bladder and bowel). Some babies will also have hydrocephalus (fluid on the brain) which can cause learning difficulties. Skin problems and latex allergies are further problems associated with spina bifida.

Conventional Medical Treatment: Initially, surgery will be required to repair the spine. This surgery needs to occur within 48 hours of birth and will repair the defect but not the nerve damage. Further treatment will depend on where the gap occurred. Physiotherapy and mobility aids can aid the child with becoming stronger and moving independently. Further orthopaedic surgery may be required if there are problems with bone development and additional treatment may be required for bowel or bladder issues. If the child has hydrocephalus, surgery will be required to insert a shunt to drain the excess fluid away to another part of the body. This shunt will usually remain in place for life.

Prognosis: A life-long condition. If treated correctly and coupled with the right support, many children live into adulthood.

Holistic Advice: When trying to get pregnant and during pregnancy ensure adequate folic acid intake. Maintain a healthy weight and eat a regular, balanced diet.

Spinal Cord Injury

Definition: Damage to the spinal cord through trauma, infection or disease.

Possible Causes: Spinal cord injuries are commonly caused by traumatic injury (e.g. fall, car accident, sports injury) and can also occur due to illness or disease. Rare neurological disorders such as transverse myelitis and Cauda Equina syndrome can both cause injury to the middle/lower areas of spinal cord. Non-malignant tumours can press on the spinal cord. Birth defects such as spina bifida are also a cause of spinal cord injury.

General Signs and Symptoms: Symptoms are dependent on the severity and location of the damage. Spinal cord injuries are often referred to as complete (no function/sensation below injury) or incomplete (some function/sensation below injury). Generally, the higher up the damage occurs the more movement and sensation is affected; however, this can vary from person to person. Damage to the spinal cord in the back can result in paraplegia where movement/sensation in the legs and sometimes the stomach muscles is affected. Damage to the spinal cord in the neck can result in tetraplegia, affecting all four limbs as well as the stomach and chest muscles. In both cases, bladder and bowel control as well as sexual function can be affected.

Conventional Medical Treatment: Dependent on the cause, location and severity. Surgery may be required to stabilise the spine after traumatic injury. Any infection will be treated with antibiotics. Enforced bed rest is most commonly required to allow the spinal cord to recover as much as possible. When on bed rest, physiotherapists will help to keep the body moving and help with any breathing difficulties. Psychological support is important to help cope with pain management and emotions following injury.

Prognosis: A life-long injury with the effects on day-to-day life dependent on the cause, location and severity. Long-term wheelchair use may be required.

Holistic Advice: Make contact with spinal cord injury organisations. Set realistic goals. Talk to family and friends about feelings and concerns.

Spinal Disorders

General Information: The spine protects the spinal cord and normally forms a straight, vertical line when viewed from the back. When viewed from the side, it has 2 main curves. It curves outwards at the top of the spine and inwards in the lower back. Abnormal curvatures of the spine can limit mobility and severely affect posture which, in turn, puts additional strain on other parts of the body. People with abnormal curvatures have a predisposition to other spinal problems later in life such as prolapsed discs. Posture can often be improved by physiotherapy, which strengthens the muscles supporting the spine. Three common spinal disorders are summarised below:

Kyphosis: Excessive outward curvature at the top of the spine. This results in a rounded back or "hunchback". The cause is not known in childhood but, in adults, disorders that limit mobility, such as osteoarthritis, or those that weaken the vertebrae, such as osteoporosis, are the most common causes. It may also be caused by poor posture (excessive slouching or leaning back in chairs) and regularly carrying heavy bags. Kyphosis can also develop as a result of injury to the spine.

Lordosis: Excessive inward curvature in the lower back. This shows as a hollow back. Lordosis may develop in those with weak abdominal muscles and poor posture. Those who are overweight are at risk of lordosis because they tend to lean back to improve balance. Kyphosis can lead to lordosis, because the lower spine compensates for the imbalance caused by the curve at the top. Kyphosis and lordosis commonly occur together, resulting in an excessive curvature at both the top of the back and in the lower back.

Scoliosis: Abnormal sideways curvature of the spine. It most commonly affects the spine in the chest area and lower back. It is more common in females and if left untreated the deformity can worsen. Scoliosis cannot be prevented and the cause is often unknown but it can be familial and in some cases the scoliosis is congenital. It can be due to skeletal defects such as unequal leg length or, rarely, muscle weakness around the spine or a neuromuscular disease. If there is no underlying cause and the scoliosis is slight, the condition will be monitored. In severe cases a spinal brace may be required to limit further curvature and surgery may be required to fuse the affected vertebrae or to straighten the spine with metal rods and wires.

Spinal Stenosis

Definition: Narrowing of the spinal canal.

Possible Causes: Most commonly caused by age related wear and tear to the bones and tissue of the spinal column. It mostly affects the lower back but can also affect the neck.

General Signs and Symptoms: Spinal stenosis may not always cause symptoms. As narrowing progresses, the nerves in the spine can become compressed. In the lower back this can lead to pain, numbness, muscle weakness and tingling in one or both legs. Walking often aggravates symptoms and causes further pain and discomfort to the point where activity will need to stop. If present in the neck, pain and weakness in the shoulders and arms might occur.

Conventional Medical Treatment: Treatment aims to relieve symptoms. Painkillers such as paracetamol and ibuprofen can be used to treat pain. Neuropathic pain medication be prescribed to help with nerve pain. Steroid injections into the spinal root canal may be recommended if other painkillers aren't sufficient. Surgery such as lumbar decompression is a last resort if symptoms are severe.

Prognosis: There is no cure but treatment can help improve symptoms. Without treatment, symptoms often gradually get worse.

Holistic Advice: Maintain a healthy weight and take regular gentle exercise.

Sprains and Strains

Definition: A sprain is a stretched, twisted or torn ligament. A strain is a stretch or tear of a muscle.

Possible Causes: Injury, commonly sustained playing sport, in which the ligament or muscle is over-stretched and damaged.

General Signs and Symptoms: Sprains cause inflammation, pain and bruising around a joint. It may not be possible to put weight on the joint and its movement may be limited. The bruising may not appear immediately and when it does may be some distance from the injured joint. Strains are graded on severity (grade 1 mild, grade 2 moderate and grade 3 severe) and cause pain, swelling and bruising in the affected muscle. A grade 3 muscle strain is also known as a rupture. This is when the muscle is torn from the tendon or the muscle itself is torn in two. This can cause the muscle to lose strength and function with severe swelling and bruising.

Conventional Medical Treatment: Usually treated from home, following the PRICE guidelines – protection, rest, ice, compression and elevation. In the case of sprains, it is considered of benefit to gently move the joint when the inflammation allows. With muscle strains, the muscle should be kept as still as possible for the first few days. Painkillers can be used to treat the pain. Surgery may be required for grade 3 strains to repair the ruptured muscle. Physiotherapy is an option post-surgery in order to return to normal activity.

Prognosis: Most sprains and strains will heal successfully. If the symptoms do not improve after a few days, medical attention should be sought.

Holistic Advice: Sprains and strains can be avoided to some extent by stretching and strengthening exercises. Warm up properly before exercise and strap weak joints. Use the correct footwear for the activity. Take rest days especially if experiencing muscular fatigue.

Stomach Cancer

Definition: Cancer found anywhere in the stomach. Also known as gastric cancer. Adenocarcinoma is the most common type in the UK and is covered below.

Possible Causes: Causes of stomach cancer are not always clear. Long term Helicobacter pylori (H. pylori) infection is a risk factor for stomach cancer. Other stomach conditions such as chronic severe acid reflux, gastritis and pernicious anaemia all increase the chances of developing stomach cancer. Lifestyle factors play a large role including smoking, being overweight or obese, alcohol consumption and working with particular chemicals can all increase risk. Men who are aged over 50 are more likely to develop the disease. Family history of the disease is also a risk factor.

General Signs and Symptoms: Symptoms can be varied and nonspecific including dysphagia (difficulty swallowing), weight loss, indigestion that will not go away, feeling full quickly, nausea, vomiting and tiredness. There may also be a lump or pain at the top of the stomach area.

Conventional Medical Treatment: Treatment dependent on the type, location, size and if it has spread to other parts of the body. If the cancer is only present in the stomach, surgery may be recommended to remove the stomach lining or part/all of the stomach (partial or total gastrectomy). Radiotherapy and chemotherapy can also be used to kill cancer cells and stop them coming back. Targeted cancer drugs such as can be prescribed to help the body control the cancerous cell growth in some circumstances.

Prognosis: Dependent on the type and stage of the cancer as well as the general health of the person. Complications can occur due to the cancer such as difficulty eating and also due to the treatment received.

Holistic Advice: Stop smoking and lose weight if required. Eat a healthy balanced diet and reduce alcohol consumption. Reduce salt and processed meat intake.

Stroke

Definition: Damage to a part of the brain caused by an interruption in its blood supply.

Possible Causes: There are 2 main causes of a stroke. The most common is when a blood clot prevents blood from reaching the brain. This is called an ischaemic stroke. Risk factors include smoking, hypertension, obesity, high cholesterol level, diabetes, irregular heartbeat, family history of heart disease or diabetes, and drinking alcohol to excess. The term "transient ischaemic attack" (TIA) is given to a temporary interruption to the blood supply to the brain. These are often a warning signs that a full blown ischemic stroke is imminent. The other main type of stoke is a haemorrhagic stroke. In this case the stroke is caused by a blood vessel in the brain bursting. Risk factors include being overweight, lack of exercise, smoking, drinking too much alcohol, taking anticoagulant medication and head injury.

General Signs and Symptoms: Signs and symptoms vary from person to person but the crucial signs can be remembered by the acronym FAST:-
F – Face: may drop on one side, person unable to smile
A – Arms: may be unable to raise (or hold up for long) one or both arms
S – Speech: may be slurred or garbled
T - Time: to dial 999 – a stroke should be considered a medical emergency
There may also be numbness on one side of the body, clumsiness, visual disturbances, headache and vomiting.

Conventional Medical Treatment: The sooner a stroke can be diagnosed and the treatment started the greater the chance of a full recovery. For ischaemic strokes, medication is given to try to dissolve the clot. Anticoagulants may be used to help prevent further clots forming. Medications can be used to help reduce the risk factors by reducing blood pressure and bringing down cholesterol levels. Emergency surgery is often required for haemorrhagic strokes to remove the leaked blood and repair the damaged vessel. Physiotherapy may be required if the stroke has caused mobility problems. Some stoke victims are left with permanent disability and may require long-term nursing care.

Prognosis: Stokes are largely avoidable by making life changes. Most stroke victims make a full recovery but about a third is left with long term disability.

Holistic Advice: Eat a healthy, low fat diet, take regular exercise, reduce stress, give up smoking and do not drink alcohol to excess.

Sunburn

Definition: Redness and swelling of the skin from overexposure to ultraviolet (UV) radiation.

Possible Causes: Sunburn is primarily caused by UV-A and UV-B radiation from the sun. Artificial UV light sources can also cause sunburn and include tanning beds. UV-A radiation penetrates the dermis, causing damage to the site the produces new skin cells. UV-B radiation causes the characteristic redness associated with sunburn. UV radiation is at its highest between 10am - 2pm with clear skies, high altitude and environmental reflection of UV radiation all contributing to an increased risk of sunburn. People with fairer or lighter skin tones are more at risk of sunburn.

General Signs and Symptoms: Dependent on skin tone and length of exposure. Typically signs and symptoms occur after exposure and are characterised by redness, swelling, tenderness and pain. The area may also feel hot to the touch. In severe cases the skin may blister and be accompanied by symptoms of fever. The skin of the affected area may begin to shed or peel off 4 – 7 days after exposure.

Conventional Medical Treatment: Treatment aims to relief discomfort. 'After sun' moisturisers and topical products containing aloe vera can be used to soothe and cool the skin. Painkillers may be used to treat pain and fever.

Prognosis: Prevention is better than cure. Chronic overexposure to UV radiation can cause premature skin ageing, brown spots and freckles. Blistering increasing the likelihood of developing skin cancers such as melanoma, basal cell carcinoma and squamous cell carcinoma. Severe cases of sunburn can result in secondary infection or death.

Holistic Advice: Wear and reapply high factor sun cream. Limit or avoid sun exposure between 10am and 2pm. Wear protective clothing such as a brimmed hat.

Superficial Thrombophlebitis

Definition: Inflammation of a vein, commonly a varicose vein, just below the surface of the skin that causes a blood clot. (Note: thrombus = blood clot, phlebitis = inflammation of a vein)

Possible Causes: Venous inflammation and the subsequent blood clot can be caused by damage to the vein, the slow flow of the blood, or blood that clots more readily than it should. Risk factors include varicose veins, long periods of inactivity, oral contraceptive pill, pregnancy, diabetes, liver disease, immunosuppressant medicines, surgery, intravenous drug injections, history of thrombosis, and cancer. This condition is more common in adult women and there could be a familial link.

General Signs and Symptoms: The skin overlying a vein may appear red, or a superficial vein may feel painful, tender, swollen and feel hard. A mild fever may be experienced. Although it can be painful, this condition is less serious than deep vein thrombosis. However, if the symptoms significantly worsen, and swelling or heat spreads up the leg, medical attention should be sought urgently.

Conventional Medical Treatment: Most cases improve in a few days without treatment. Painkillers may be used to treat the pain and the leg may feel more comfortable rested and raised. Compression stockings can help. If the condition is caused by the blood clotting too readily, anticoagulants may be prescribed. If a varicose vein causes repeated problems it may be removed.

Prognosis: Rarely it may spread up to a deep vein, leading to deep vein thrombosis.

Holistic Advice: Take regular gentle exercise, do not smoke and try to avoid getting varicose veins.

<u>Sycosis Barbae</u>

Definition: Bacterial infection and subsequent inflammation of the hair follicles of the beard.

Possible Causes: Begins as a bacterial infection called folliculitis barbae caused by the staphylococcus aureus bacteria when it enters the hair follicle, most commonly after shaving. When this condition progresses deeper in the hair follicle and to adjoining follicles it is known as sycosis barbae. Those who suffer with sinusitis and hay fever are susceptible to reoccurring infections as staphylococcus aureus lives in the nose.

General Signs and Symptoms: Large red regions and swollen lumps (similar to boils) on the beard area. Discharge, pus, tenderness and pain may also be present.

Conventional Medical Treatment: Dependent on severity. Oral and topical antibiotics are the primary treatment for the bacterial infection. Steroid creams may be prescribed to reduce inflammation.

Prognosis: Most cases clear after treatment. Severe infections can cause scarring, hair loss and abscesses. Without treatment infection may spread.

Holistic Advice: Prevention is key. Adopt good shaving practices (e.g. use a sharp razor), or, alternatively look for longer-term methods of hair removal such as laser or electrolysis.

Syphilis

Definition: A bacterial infection.

Possible Causes: Caused by Treponema pallidum bacteria. It is usually caught via sexual intercourse with an infected person. It is also possible to catch syphilis if you share a needle with an infected person. Infected pregnant women can pass it to their unborn baby.

General Signs and Symptoms: Initial symptoms start 2 – 3 weeks after infection and pass within 2 – 8 weeks. These include a small painless sore(s) on the genitals, anus or mouth and swollen glands in the neck, groin or armpits. If the infection is not treated secondary syphilis can develop including symptoms such as blotchy red rash on the palms of hands or soles of feet, small skin growths on the genitals or anus, patchy hair loss and flu like symptoms such as lethargy, headache, joint pain, fever and swollen glands.

Conventional Medical Treatment: Type of treatment dependent on how long the person has had the infection. It is usually treated with a short course of antibiotics administered either via injection into the buttocks or with tablets. Pregnant women can also be safety treated with antibiotics. Any sexual partners since infection of will also need to be tested and treated.

Prognosis: Infection persists even if symptoms disappear. When treated with antibiotics common side effects are flu like symptoms (fever, headache and muscle/joint pain). If left untreated for a long time (years), syphilis can spread to the brain causing long-term issues including meningitis, stroke, dementia symptoms, numbness, vision loss and heart problems.

Holistic Advice: Prevention is key; use of a condom or barrier during sexual intercourse or oral sex is recommended to prevent infection. Avoid sharing sex toys. Avoid sex during treatment.

Tendonitis

Definition: Inflammation of a tendon.

Possible Causes: Overuse of a tendon or injury, often in the shoulder, elbow (tennis elbow), wrist, fingers, thigh, knee, or back of heel. It is more common in sportsmen, due to the risk of overuse and injury, and in the elderly because tendons become less elastic with age. Tendonitis is also more common in people with diabetes.

General Signs and Symptoms: Pain, a grating or cracking sensation, swelling, and weakness in the affected area. A lump may develop along the tendon.

Conventional Medical Treatment: Painkillers and ice/heat packs will usually be sufficient. Steroid injections and physiotherapy can also be used. If calcium deposits have built up around the tendon (calcific tendonitis), they can be removed surgically or treated with shock waves.

Prognosis: Episodes usually only last a few days but can be more persistent.

Holistic Advice: Rest the tendon during an episode. Avoid repetitive movement and exercise the affected area to strengthen the muscles around the tendon to try to avoid another episode. Warm up before exercise and cool down properly after it.

Tennis Elbow / Golfers Elbow

Definition: Inflammation of a tendon (tendonitis) at its attachment to the bone at the elbow. Tennis elbow affects the outside of the elbow and golfer's elbow affects the inner side of the elbow. Tennis elbow is referred to as lateral epicondylitis and golfer's elbow is called medial epicondylitis.

Possible Causes: Vigorous and/or repeated use of muscles in the forearm can damage the muscles and tendons. Common activities that cause overuse and hence tennis or golfer's elbow include racquet sports, sports involving throwing, swimming, and the extensive use of gardening shears. It can also be brought on by work that involves repetitive wrist action (e.g. brick laying and typing).

General Signs and Symptoms: Pain and tenderness on the outside of the elbow (tennis elbow) or the inner side (golfer's elbow). The pain may radiate down the forearm and twisting movements are often particularly painful. Repetitive wrist movements can make the pain worse. The pain may range from mild when the joint is moved, to severe pain even at rest.

Conventional Medical Treatment: Anti-inflammatory drugs can be used for the pain and, in severe cases, a corticosteroid injection may be recommended. Physiotherapy may be required to help stretch and strengthen the muscles in the forearm. Surgery can be used but only usually as a last resort.

Prognosis: In most cases the symptoms eventually clear up without treatment but tendons are slow to heal and so this may take several weeks, months or even over a year.

Holistic Advice: Try to limit the chance of damaging the tendons by warming up properly before playing sport, seek advice on sporting technique, and try to avoid movements that cause pain. Rest a painful arm as soon as possible. Ice packs may bring relief. Acupuncture claims to be effective in some cases.

Testicular Cancer

Definition: Cancer of the testicle. Two most common types are seminomas and non-seminomas. Less common types are Leydig cell tumours and Sertoli cell tumours.

Possible Causes: The exact causes of testicular cancer are unknown but there are many risk factors that are thought to increase the chance of developing it. These risk factors include undescended testicles, family history of testicular cancer and previous diagnosis of testicular cancer.

General Signs and Symptoms: Only a very small minority of lumps or swelling are cancerous. Typically a painless swelling or lump in one of the testicles develops, often the size of a pea. Symptoms can also include any change in shape or texture of testicle such as increase in firmness. Sometimes intermittent sharp pain or dull ache in the testicle or scrotum is felt.

Conventional Medical Treatment: Dependent on the type and stage of cancer. For all cases the first treatment option is to surgically remove the testicle affected. A combination of chemotherapy and radiotherapy might offered after surgery. Testosterone replacement therapy can be offered if the remaining healthy testicle is not making enough.

Prognosis: Removing the entire affected testicle greatly enhances the chance of a full recovery. Fertility and sex life should not be affected however there is a chance that aggressive treatment will cause fertility issues such as a low sperm count. There is a chance that the cancer will return in the other testicle in the future. If both testicles are removed then infertility will occur.

Holistic Advice: Check the testicles regularly for any signs of lumps or changes in appearance. See a GP as soon as possible if you notice any changes. Be extra vigilant if you have family history of testicular cancer.

Testicular Lumps (Benign)

Definition: A variety of non-cancerous lumps that may form in the testes. There are 4 main types of benign testicular lump - varicocele, hydrocele, epididymal cyst and testicular torsion.

Possible Causes: Varicocele is a collection of varicose veins in the scrotum, possibly caused by abnormalities in the veins (including weakened valves) that results in a swelling due to the accumulation of blood. Hydrocele is the accumulation of fluid in the scrotum. In adult men this may be caused by infection, inflammation or injury of the testis. An epididymal cyst is a fluid-filled swelling caused by the accumulation of skin cells and protein. A testicular torsion is caused when the testis twists on the spermatic cord within the scrotum, often interrupting the blood supply.

General Signs and Symptoms: Many lumps cause no other symptoms but are discovered by routine examinations. Others may cause a heavy sensation or pain in the scrotum or groin. Varicoceles tend not to cause any symptoms other than the swelling, develop on the left side of the scrotum and may feel like a bag of worms. Hydroceles are only evident by the swelling although the fluid may cause the scrotum to feel heavy. Epididymal cysts may become infected, in which case they can become red, painful and smelly. Testicular tortion is extremely painful and is a medical emergency. If not treated very quickly the testis may have to be removed. Sudden pain in the scrotum, groin and lower abdomen, redness and extreme tenderness of the scrotum, nausea, vomiting and a fever are typical symptoms.

Conventional Medical Treatment: Small varicoceles do not usually need to be treated and often disappear. If surgery is required the procedure is to inject the veins with a chemical that causes the veins to block. Hydroceles only tend to be treated if they are causing problems in which case the fluid is drained from the scrotum. Epididymal cysts normally remain small and do not require treatment. If they become infected corticosteroid injections can be used or they can be surgically removed. Testicular torsion is corrected by surgery.

Prognosis: With the exception of testicular torsion, benign testicular lumps do not tend to have any associated complications.

Holistic Advice: All men should be encouraged to examine their testicles regularly. Only about 4% of all testicular lumps are malignant but it is important to get a diagnosis if any testicular lump is found. Testicular cancer is one of the most easily treated cancers if detected early.

Tetanus

Definition: A bacterial infection that produces severe muscle stiffness and spasms. It is quite rare in developed countries because most people have now been immunized. Commonly called lockjaw.

Possible Causes: Caused by the Clostridium tetani bacterium, which lives in soil, dust and the manure of animals such as horses and cows. The bacteria enter the body through open wounds. Once in the body they multiply, releasing a neurotoxin. The neurotoxin is carried around the body in the bloodstream, blocking nerve impulses from the spinal cord to the muscles. There is a risk of infection when the skin is damaged by burns, and the infection can also be introduced to the body by animal bites, body piercing, tattoos, intravenous drug use etc.

General Signs and Symptoms: Symptoms develop about 10 days after infection and are typified by muscle stiffness (particularly in the face and jaws) and painful muscle spasms (particularly in the neck, throat and face). There may also be a fever, headache, rapid heart beat and hypertension. If the muscles of the throat or chest are affected it can lead to problems swallowing and breathing difficulties respectively. Spasms in the back can cause the spine to arch backwards.

Conventional Medical Treatment: Immediate treatment is required. Antitoxin injections and antibiotics may be used. Sedatives may be needed to relieve any muscle spasms.

Prognosis: If the infection is not treated immediately it can be fatal.

Holistic Advice: Keep tetanus vaccine up to date, especially if travelling or in contact with soil and manure (e.g. farming and gardening). Wash any wounds and treat them with antiseptic immediately. If not vaccinated, see a Doctor with any wounds contaminated with soil or manure or with any deep wounds.

Thalassaemia

Definition: A group of inherited conditions that affect the level of haemoglobin in the blood. The two most common types of thalassaemia are alpha and beta. These types can be further categorised as minor or major depending on the number of genes affected. Beta thalassaemia major is the most severe.

Possible Causes: Thalassaemia is caused by a faulty gene and inherited genetically. The parents may not have thalassaemia themselves, but just carry the faulty gene that causes it. Those at most risk include people from or with family from the Mediterranean, India, Pakistan, Bangladesh, the Middle East, China and southeast Asia.

General Signs and Symptoms: The most common condition to develop is anaemia due to low levels of haemoglobin (the substance that transports oxygen) in the blood. This is characterised by tiredness, shortness of breath, heart palpitations, pale skin and jaundice. Those with thalassaemia major may experience a build-up of iron in the body causing heart problems, swelling of the liver (cirrhosis), delayed puberty, low levels of sex hormones (oestrogen and testosterone), diabetes and problems with the thyroid and parathyroid glands. Thalassaemia major can also cause gallstones, unusual bone growth, osteoporosis and reduced fertility. Children born with beta thalassaemia major will most likely develop symptoms shortly after birth. Less severe types may not experience symptoms until late childhood or early adulthood.

Conventional Medical Treatment: Usually requires lifelong treatment and depends on the type and severity. For severe types, regular blood transfusions, around once a month, will be required to treat anaemia. Less severe types will only need them occasionally. Chelation therapy is used to remove excess iron from the blood caused by regular blood transfusions.

Prognosis: Usually requires lifelong management and treatment. Extra precautions should be taken when going under general anaesthetic.

Holistic Advice: Eat a healthy balanced diet and exercise regularly. Avoid smoking and limit alcohol consumption. Practice good hand hygiene to reduce risk of infection.

Thrush (Vaginal)

Definition: Inflammation and irritation of the vagina and vulva caused by a fungal infection.

Possible Causes: Caused by a Candida fungal infection, most commonly the Candida albicans fungus. The Candida fungus lives naturally in the vagina without causing any problems but then conditions change and thrush is triggered. Risk factors include taking antibiotics, pregnancy, diabetes and a damaged immune system. Stress, sexual activity, tight fitting clothing, and the combined oral contraceptive pill may also be contributory triggers.

General Signs and Symptoms: Intense irritation and itching of the vagina and vulva, pain or discomfort during sex and urination, and there may be a vaginal discharge.

Conventional Medical Treatment: Anti-fungal medications can be taken either orally or inserted into the vagina. Topical creams can help soothe sore parts of the genitals.

Prognosis: Treatment is usually effective but the infection can recur.

Holistic Advice: Avoid perfumed soap or other scented products that may come into contact with the genitals, keep the genitals clean, dry and cool, wear loose fitting clothing and cotton underwear, wipe the bottom from front to back after going to the toilet, reduce stress, and avoid sex until the condition has cleared. Make sure the vagina is well lubricated before sexual intercourse, but avoid latex condoms, spermicidal creams and lubricants if they are found to cause irritation. Boost the immune system.

Thyroid Cancer

Definition: Cancer found in the thyroid, a butterfly shaped gland at the front of the neck.

Possible Causes: Exact cause is unknown but women are more likely to develop thyroid cancer than men. Risk factors include having other conditions such as thyroiditis, Hashimoto's disease, systemic lupus erythematosus, goitre (enlarged thyroid), familial adenomatous polyposis and acromegaly. A family history of thyroid cancer and previous radiotherapy treatment can also increase the risk of developing the disease. Lifestyle factors such as being overweight or obese are also risk factors.

General Signs and Symptoms: The main symptoms include a lump at the front of the neck, a persistent sore throat and a persistent hoarse voice. Difficulty swallowing, difficulty breathing and pain in the neck may also be experienced. If the cancer affects the production of the thyroid hormones diarrhoea and flushing may occur.

Conventional Medical Treatment: Treatment dependent on the location, size and type of the cancer. Surgery to remove part or the entire thyroid is the most common treatment option. Radioactive iodine treatment, external radiotherapy, chemotherapy and targeted therapies may be used to kill cancer cells.

Prognosis: Dependent on the location, size and type of the cancer. If part or all of the thyroid is removed medication will be needed to replace the missing hormones. Calcium supplements may be required if the parathyroid glands are affected during surgery. Surgery to remove part or all of the thyroid may cause damage to the voice box.

Holistic Advice: Lose weight (if required).

Tonsillitis

Definition: Inflammation of the tonsils.

Possible Causes: Can be caused by either a bacterial or, most commonly, a viral infection. Bacterial tonsillitis is likely to be caused by group A streptococcus bacteria. Viruses that affect the respiratory system, including the flu virus, are usually the ones responsible for viral tonsillitis. The Epstein-Barr virus that causes glandular fever can also cause tonsillitis.

General Signs and Symptoms: Sore throat, red, swollen tonsils, white pus-filled spots on the tonsils, pain when swallowing, fever, coughing, headache, tiredness and swollen lymph glands in the neck.

Conventional Medical Treatment: If the tonsillitis is caused by a bacterial infection antibiotics can be used. Painkillers, lozenges and throat sprays can help ease the symptoms. Tonsillectomy can be undertaken to remove the tonsils in severe or recurring cases.

Prognosis: Usually clears up on its own but in severe or recurring cases the tonsils can be removed.

Holistic Advice: Drink plenty of fluids and try to eat. Boost the immune system.

Toothache

Definition: Pain or discomfort in one or more teeth or in the gums.

Possible Causes: Toothache can be caused by many disorders of the teeth including dental decay, cavities, tooth fractures, pulpitis (inflammation of the pulp in the tooth) receding gums and abscesses. Pain may also arise from teeth that are misaligned.

General Signs and Symptoms: Pain in a tooth and/or gum that may radiate to the face, neck and ears. The pain may be worse when chewing or if the teeth are exposed to heat or cold. There may be a swelling around the affected tooth and the tooth or gums may bleed. Toothache over a period of time can affect nutrition and can be very wearing.

Conventional Medical Treatment: The treatment will depend on the cause of the pain. X-rays can help determine the extent of the problem. The tooth may be filled, capped or removed. Abscesses may be treated with antibiotics and/or drained. Root canal treatment, in which the decayed area, pulp cavity and root canals are filled, may be required if the decay invades the pulp. Painkillers can be used to help relieve the pain. Orthodontic treatments can be used to correct crowded or unevenly spaced teeth.

Prognosis: Not usually considered to be serious however, if left untreated, the infection from an abscess can spread into the bone and bloodstream causing serious complications.

Holistic Advice: Cut down on sugary foods, thoroughly brush the teeth at least twice a day, use dental floss and mouthwash to help clean between the teeth, don't smoke and visit a dentist annually for a check up.

Toxic Shock Syndrome (TSS)

Definition: Life-threatening condition caused by bacteria releasing harmful toxins into the body

Possible Causes: Often associated with tampon use in women but can affect anyone, of any age. TSS is caused by either staphylococcus or streptococcus bacteria. Risk factors that increase the chance of getting TSS are; using tampons (especially if left in longer than advised), using female barrier contraceptives such as the diaphragm or cap, a problem cut, burn, boil, insect bite or surgery wound, childbirth and contracting either staphylococcus or streptococcus infections (e.g. throat infection, impetigo or cellulitis).

General Signs and Symptoms: Start suddenly and get worse very quickly. Including; high temperature, flu-like symptoms (headache, lethargy, aching, sore throat, cough), nausea, vomiting, diarrhoea, widespread sunburn-like rash, dizziness/fainting, difficulty breathing, confusion and the lips/tongue/whites of eyes turning bright red.

Conventional Medical Treatment: Admittance into hospital and sometimes intensive care to receive treatment that may involve; antibiotics, oxygen, fluids for dehydration, medicine to control blood pressure, dialysis if the kidneys are affected. In severe cases, surgery or amputation might be necessary to remove dead tissue.

Prognosis: TSS is a medical emergency and immediate medical advice should be sought. If diagnosed quickly and treated early most people make a full recovery. With quick treatment, most people will start to recover within a few days though it could be several weeks until the person is well enough to leave hospital.

Holistic Advice: Treat wounds/burns quickly and seek medical advice if there are any signs of infection. Practice good hand hygiene before/after inserting a tampon, change the tampon regularly, and always use a tampon with the lowest absorbency level for your period. Alternate between tampons, sanitary towel or panty liners during your period.

Tracheitis

Definition: Inflammation of the trachea (windpipe) due to infection. A rare condition that typically affects young children.

Possible Causes: Most commonly caused by the Staphylococcus aureus bacteria. Although rare, most cases occur after an initial upper respiratory tract infection (such as a common cold) where the bacteria can more easily gain access to the trachea.

General Signs and Symptoms: After initial cold symptoms (cough, runny/blocked nose) signs of infection will develop. These include high fever, difficulty breathing, wheezing and a deeper, stronger cough. Stridor (high-pitched sound when breathing) may also be developed. This is a sign that the airway is being obstructed by inflammation and is often confused with croup.

Conventional Medical Treatment: Initial treatment with antibiotics, usually given intravenously. If the airway is blocked substantially the child may be intubated and ventilated whilst they recover from the infection.

Prognosis: Dependant on severity but usually once over the acute infection the majority of children recover fully. Speed of treatment is very important to a full recovery. If caused by the Staphylococcus aureus bacteria there is a small chance of toxic shock syndrome developing.

Holistic Advice: Look at boosting the immune system.

Trichomonas

Definition: A parasitic sexually transmitted infection.

Possible Causes: Caused by the trichomonas vaginalis (TV) parasite caught via unprotected sexual intercourse. It can also be spread by sharing sex toys with an infected person.

General Signs and Symptoms: Usually develop within 1 month of infection but often no symptoms are displayed at all. In women, the infection affects the vagina and urethra and can cause abnormal vaginal discharge (including a change in colour, unpleasant smell or producing more than usual), soreness, swelling or itchiness around the vagina and pain when urinating or having sex. In men the infection commonly affects the urethra but infection can also reach the head of the penis and prostate gland. Symptoms can include pain when urinating or ejaculating, increased urination, thin, white discharge from the penis and soreness/swelling around the head of the penis.

Conventional Medical Treatment: Effectively treated with a short course of antibiotics. Current and recent sexual partners should also be tested and treated.

Prognosis: Infection persists even if symptoms are not present. Complications are rare. If infected whilst pregnant the infection can spread to the baby, which can cause premature birth and low birth weight.

Holistic Advice: Prevention is key; use of a condom or barrier during sexual intercourse. Avoid sharing sex toys, if you do share them ensure they are covered with a condom and cleaned after use.

Tuberculosis

Definition: A bacterial infection that most often affects the lungs but can affect other parts of the body. Often abbreviated to TB.

Possible Causes: Caused by the bacteria Mycobacterium tuberculosis and it is spread through the droplets of saliva dispersed by the coughs and sneezes of an infected person. In many healthy people the infection is fought off and the bacteria killed by the immune system and so the condition does not progress. In others, the TB bacteria may lie dormant and reactivate years later if the person's immunity is reduced. People with reduced immunity are at greatest risk from developing TB, e.g those with HIV, diabetes mellitus or taking immunosuppressant drugs. Other risk factors include long term lung disease, living in overcrowded conditions with poor sanitation, traveling to parts of the world where TB is more prevalent, the elderly and the very young.

General Signs and Symptoms: Initially there may be no symptoms until a cough develops and the infected person feels generally unwell. If the disease progresses the cough becomes persistent and productive, and there may be chest pain on deep inhalation, shortness of breath, fever, poor appetite, weight loss, night sweats and tiredness. If the infection spreads to other parts of the body additional symptoms are caused. Rarely the infection does not begin in the lungs, for example if unpasteurised milk is drunk from a cow infected with TB, the infection may begin in the gastrointestinal tract.

Conventional Medical Treatment: Can usually be treated effectively with a combination of oral antituberculous drugs (antibiotics) taken for about 6 months. The BCG vaccine against TB is available.

Prognosis: Left untreated it may cause long term illness and death. Some types of TB are more resistant to the drugs than others. Even treated the disease can still be fatal in those whose immunity is severely weakened.

Holistic Advice: Boost the immune system. If infected, try to prevent the spread of the disease by taking care when coughing, disposing of tissues carefully and maintaining good hand hygiene.

Ulcerative Colitis

Definition: Chronic intermittent inflammation and ulceration of the colon.

Possible Causes: The lining of the colon becomes inflamed, swollen and ulcerates. The ulcers can bleed and create mucus and pus. The exact cause is unknown but there may possibly be genetic and environmental links. Some believe that it may be caused by a malfunction in the immune system. Tends to develop in young adults.

General Signs and Symptoms: Diarrhoea (often containing blood and mucus), abdominal pain, tiredness, loss of appetite, weight loss, anaemia, fever, a constant need to open the bowels, and dehydration. Symptoms can range from mild to severe and the number of attacks can vary.

Conventional Medical Treatment: Mild-moderate cases can usually be successfully treated with drugs. Aminosalicylates (to reduce inflammation), steroids (if aminosalicylates are not strong enough) and immunosuppressants (also to help reduce the inflammation) can be prescribed. Surgery to remove the colon may be required. This results in a colostomy (the creation of a stoma in the abdominal wall through which faeces is passed).

Prognosis: Can usually be successfully managed but complications can arise in severe cases. Sufferers of ulcerative colitis have an increased risk of colorectal cancer. This risk increases with the length of time the condition has been present.

Holistic Advice: Keep a diary to see if any foods worsen the condition. Drink plenty of fluids. Try to reduce stress levels.

Uraemia

Definition: Build-up of urea in the blood, a major symptom of kidney failure.

Possible Causes: Uraemia occurs when the kidneys have become seriously damaged, often beyond repair. This is often due to chronic kidney disease.

General Signs and Symptoms: Uraemia can cause symptoms such as extreme tiredness/fatigue, leg cramps, loss of appetite, headache, nausea and vomiting.

Conventional Medical Treatment: The main form of treatment for uraemia is dialysis, which is used to artificially filter the blood. If the person is suffering from kidney failure then kidney transplant is another possible treatment option.

Prognosis: If dialysis appointments are consistently attended then uraemia should be reduced or stopped altogether. Can be fatal if left untreated.

Holistic Advice: Control diabetes and maintain a healthy blood pressure. Stop smoking and take regular exercise. Avoid foods high in salt and potassium.

Urinary Incontinence

Definition: The complete or partial loss of voluntary control over bladder function. There are four types. 1. Stress incontinence, which is the involuntary loss of urine during exertion. 2. Urge incontinence, which is characterized by repeated episodes of involuntary loss of urine preceded by a sudden and urgent need to empty the bladder. 3. Overflow incontinence, in which there is often a blockage that prevents the bladder from emptying properly. The urine builds up and the pressure causes leaks. 4. Total incontinence, when there is no bladder control at all. Stress and urge are covered below, as they are the most common.

Possible Causes: Stress incontinence occurs when the pelvic floor muscles weaken to the extent that they cannot prevent urination. Pelvic muscles may weaken as a result of pregnancy, childbirth, menopause, hysterectomy, age and obesity. Urge incontinence occurs when the bladder is unstable or overactive and contracts too early, often before the bladder is full. The exact cause is unknown but it is thought to occur as a result of incorrect signals being sent between the brain and the bladder, or the irritability of the muscle in the bladder wall by infection or inflammation. Mild urinary incontinence may be triggered by some medicines (e.g. diuretics and muscle relaxants), certain drinks (e.g. alcohol, coffee (both diuretics), citrus fruit juices and drinks containing artificial sweeteners. Chronic coughing can also weaken the sphincter.

General Signs and Symptoms: The main symptom is the loss of voluntary bladder control which causes urination to take place unintentionally. Losing a small amount of urine upon activities such as coughing or sneezing is symptomatic of stress incontinence. The sudden, urgent, and usually frequent need to urinate is typical of urge incontinence. There may be only seconds between warning and urination.

Conventional Medical Treatment: The type and severity of the condition will affect the treatment. Lifestyle changes and pelvic floor exercises may help all types. For stress incontinence a number of surgical procedures are available. For urge incontinence, bladder training may help lengthen the time between feeling the need to urinate and urinating. Medication (e.g. antimuscarinics) to help relax the muscle in the bladder and surgical options are possible but not without risks.

Prognosis: Lifestyle changes may help and medical intervention can help ease the symptoms.

Holistic Advice: Reduce caffeine and alcohol intake, lose excess weight, stop smoking and ensure fluid intake is correct. This condition can be upsetting for the sufferer so remember to treat any anxiety or depression.

Urticaria

Definition: A raised itchy rash also known as hives, weals, welts or nettle rash. Urticaria can be acute (present for less than 6 weeks) or chronic (persists or reoccurs for more than 6 weeks).

Possible Causes: Urticaria occurs when high levels of histamine and other chemical messengers are released in the skin, dilating the blood vessels and allowing fluid to leak into the area. This is usually due to a specific 'trigger' though the exact cause is often unidentifiable. Triggers can include a recent acute viral or bacterial infection, a food allergy, cold or heat exposure, allergy/reaction to an insect bite/sting, medication or contact with particular plants, chemicals and latex. The exact cause of chronic urticaria is not definitive and thought to be an autoimmune reaction. It has been linked to other autoimmune conditions such as rheumatoid arthritis and lupus as well as chronic illnesses such as viral hepatitis. Triggers such as alcohol, caffeine and stress, as well as those listed above, have been shown to make chronic urticaria symptoms reappear or worsen.

General Signs and Symptoms: Characterised by raised red patches and/or spots. These hives can occur anywhere on the body, can be any size or shape and are often itchy, coupled with a burning or stinging sensation. More severe urticaria can also present with angioedema (swelling under the skin). Angioedema mostly affects the areas around the eyes and lips but can cause swelling in the upper respiratory tract.

Conventional Medical Treatment: If mild, urticaria may not require treatment. Antihistamines such as cetirizine, fexofenadine and loratadine can help with itching and reduce the rash. Oral steroids may be prescribed for more severe cases. Chronic or persistent urticaria may require referral to a dermatologist.

Prognosis: Can resolve by itself with a few minutes to a few days. Chronic urticaria can cause emotional distress and requires more careful management to identify and avoid triggers. Urticaria can be one of the first symptoms of severe allergic reaction or anaphylaxis.

Holistic Advice: Avoid known triggers and allergies. Limit alcohol and caffeine intake. Try to reduce stress levels and practice breathing or meditation techniques.

Vaginitis

Definition: Soreness and swelling in and around the vagina.

Possible Causes: There are numerous possible causes such as irritation from soap, injury to the vagina, thrush, chlamydia or trichomonas (STI's), hormonal changes from menopause, breastfeeding, some types of contraception and skin conditions like eczema.

General Signs and Symptoms: One or a combination of the following symptoms are common; sore, swollen or cracked skin around the vagina, vaginal dryness, different colour, smell or thickness of vaginal discharge, vaginal dryness and pain when urinating or having sex.

Conventional Medical Treatment: Treatment will depend on the underlying cause. For thrush, antifungal medicines will be prescribed. For an STI such as chlamydia, antibiotics. For menopause, hormone treatments and lubricants might be used and for skin conditions like eczema, steroid medicines.

Prognosis: A common condition that is easily treatable once the underlying cause has been discovered. Sometimes the condition reoccurs, depending on the cause.

Holistic Advice: Stop the use of scented hygiene products in/around the vagina and do not douche. When washing, use water and dry thoroughly. Try wearing loose cotton underwear.

Varicose Veins

Definition: Swollen and enlarged veins.

Possible Causes: Varicose veins are caused by the weakening of the valves that prevent the backflow of blood in the veins. It is not fully understood why this happens but risk factors include sex (women are more likely to suffer), prolonged standing, being overweight, age, family history of the disease and pregnancy.

General Signs and Symptoms: Dark blue/purple, lumpy, bulging veins, most commonly occurring in the calves of the legs where they are visible through the skin. Some people will not experience any discomfort as a result of the varicose veins. Others may find the legs ache, throb or cramp, and the feet and ankles may swell. The skin over the affected area may also become dry, thin and itchy and occasionally leg ulcers may arise. Varicose veins can occur in other parts of the body, e.g. oesophagus, uterus, vagina, pelvis and rectum.

Conventional Medical Treatment: Treatment will only be required if the varicose veins are causing discomfort, if they are causing complications, or for cosmetic reasons. Treatments include compression stockings, sclerotherapy (in which a chemical is injected into the vein to seal it so preventing blood from entering) or surgery to remove them.

Prognosis: Varicose veins may not look nice, but they do not usually affect circulation or create any other serious health problems. Varicose veins may recur even after surgery.

Holistic Advice: Take regular exercise such as swimming and walking to keep the blood flowing in the legs. Raise the legs when resting to aid blood flow. Avoid prolonged sitting or standing and do not cross the legs when sitting. Support stockings can be beneficial, particularly to those who have to stand a lot, and avoid wearing tight clothing that restricts the blood flow at the top of the legs. Lose excess weight and stop smoking. Never massage over or below a varicose vein.

Vitiligo

Definition: A long-term depigmenting disorder of the skin. There are two main types, non-segmental vitiligo (most common) and segmental vitiligo.

Possible Causes: Melanocytes, the cells that produce the pigment melanin, are lost or destroyed causing the colour of the skin to become progressively lighter. The exact cause of the destruction of the melanocytes is unknown but non-segmental vitiligo is thought to be an autoimmune condition. Risk factors for developing non-segmental vitiligo include family history of autoimmune conditions, having a pre-existing autoimmune condition, melanoma, non-Hodgkin lymphoma and having another family member with vitiligo. Segmental vitiligo is less common and is believed to be caused by chemicals released by the nerve endings in the skin destroying the melanocytes. There is some evidence to suggest that vitiligo can be triggered by stressful events, severe skin damage or exposure to specific chemicals.

General Signs and Symptoms: Severity differs between individuals and there is no way to predict how much pigment will be lost. Non-segmental vitiligo (bilateral or generalised vitiligo) is characterised by white patches ion the body which are often symmetrical. These symmetrical patches can occur on the arms, knees, elbows, backs of the hands/feet and the skin around the eyes. Segmental vitiligo (unilateral or localised vitiligo) only affects one area of the body. Although rare, vitiligo can affect the whole body. When this happens, it is known as universal or complete vitiligo.

Conventional Medical Treatment: Treatment aims to restore the colour of the skin. Topical steroids may reduce the spread of vitiligo and restore some of the original skin colour. Phototherapy (UV radiation) can be recommended to individuals if the vitiligo covers most of the body and topical treatments haven't worked. Stable vitiligo that hasn't changed for an extended period of time can be treated with skin grafts, dermabrasion or laser techniques. Depigmentation therapy may be recommended for individuals who have widespread vitiligo. Cosmetic camouflage products can be used to cover up patches of vitiligo. If the condition is causing distress, cognitive behavioural therapy (CBT) may be of help.

Prognosis: The effects of treatment are not often permanent and cannot guarantee to control the condition. Risk of sunburn is very high and precautions to protect the skin from the sun should be taken.

Holistic Advice: Use high factor sun cream to protect the skin. Take steps to minimise injury to the skin.

Warts / Verrucae

Definition: Small, horny, benign (non-cancerous) tumours of the skin.

Possible Causes: Human papilloma virus (HPV) causes the protein keratin in the top layer of the skin to grow too much. More common in those who have atopic eczema or weakened immune systems. Damaged and wet skin is more vulnerable.

General Signs and Symptoms: Common warts (verruca vulgaris) are rough, raised and horny commonly occurring on the hands, elbows and knees. Verrucae are called plantar warts and they are found on the sole of the foot, heels and toes. Verrucae grow into the skin rather than outwards and often have a black dot in the centre. They are more painful than other types and spread rapidly, especially in places with a humid environment such as swimming pools. Plane/flat warts (verruca plana) are round, flat-topped and usually yellowish. They usually occur in children, rarely adults. Filiform warts (verruca filiformis) are long, slender warts, commonly found on the skin of the eyelids, armpits or neck. Mosaic warts are warts that grow in clusters, mainly on the hands (palmer warts) and feet. Genital warts, found of the genitalia and anal area, is classified as a sexually transmitted disease and medical attention should be sought.

Conventional Medical Treatment: Creams, gels, paints and medicated plasters containing salicylic acid can be used topically, taking great care to avoid contact with healthy skin. They should not be used on the face without seeking medical advice and caution is required in cases of poor circulation. Covering the wart with duct tape has few side effects when the recommended program is followed. Cryotherapy involves freezing the wart using a very cold liquid such as nitrogen. This is usually undertaken in hospital skin clinics. Surgery is not common but there are other options to remove the wart using lasers, electrical current or chemicals. Do not self-treat genital warts – consult a medical practitioner.

Prognosis: Usually harmless and often clear up on own accord but treatment can speed up their removal. Warts/verrucae are contagious and so direct and indirect contact should be avoided when possible.

Holistic Advice: Warts will generally disappear as quickly as they arrive. As warts may be visible there may be associated psychological implications. As this is a viral infection, anything to boost the immune system may help. Vitamin E and a balanced diet can be of benefit. If a wart is brown, feels soft, suddenly changes its shape or appearance, itches, bleeds, produces a discharge or spreads, a GP should be consulted. There is a greater chance of a wart becoming malignant in cases of poor immune systems.

Whiplash

Definition: Spinal injury in which the ligaments, tendons and muscles of the neck are damaged by a sudden movement of the head forwards, backwards or sideways.

Possible Causes: The injury commonly occurs as a result of a road traffic incident. An impact from the rear, front or side can result in a whiplash injury. It can also be caused by a blow to the head or a fall that causes the head to jolt violently. The over-extension or over-flexion of the neck damages the muscles, tendons and ligaments. Whiplash tends to affect more women than men, probably because the neck muscles in women are not so strong.

General Signs and Symptoms: Symptoms vary according to the severity of the injury. Symptoms may include pain, stiffness, lack of movement, swelling, bruising and tenderness in the neck, lower back pain, headaches, muscle spasms, pain or numbness in the shoulders and arms, dizziness, tinnitus, blurred vision, vertigo and tiredness. There may even be some memory loss. Sometimes the symptoms can last long-term. This is called chronic whiplash. Chronic whiplash can sometimes lead to anxiety and depression.

Conventional Medical Treatment: Keeping the neck as mobile as possible is largely encouraged. Painkillers and non-steroidal anti-inflammatories can help to reduce the pain. Physiotherapy may be recommended.

Prognosis: In most acute cases the whiplash clears up with minimum treatment. The range of symptoms associated with chronic cases (lasting for more than 6 months) can be troublesome.

Holistic Advice: Maintaining a good posture and using a supportive pillow may help the healing. Exercises to strengthen the muscles may be of benefit. If the whiplash is due to an accident, there may be psychological aspects to deal with such as shock and loss of confidence. A car's headrest positioned at the correct height can help prevent the head from being whipped back should an accident occur.

Whitlow

Definition: Infection of the tip of the finger (staphylococcal whitlow) or the end of the finger (herpetic whitlow).

Possible Causes: There are two types of whitlow, staphylococcal most commonly caused by the staphylococcal aureus bacteria and herpetic caused by the herpes simplex virus type 1 (HSV-1). Staphylococcal whitlow occurs when staphylococcal aureus bacteria gain entry to the body through a break in the skin or untreated paronychia (infection of the fold of skin that surrounds the nail). Herpetic whitlow usually occurs when a person with oral herpes touches their mouth with their hands and spreads the virus via a break in the skin. Hepatic whitlow can also be spread through physical contact with a person with active oral herpes symptoms. Less commonly, herpetic whitlow can be caused and spread through contact with genital herpes (HSV-2).

General Signs and Symptoms: Staphylococcal whitlow is characterised by rapid onset of very severe throbbing pain, swelling and redness at the fingertip. Herpetic whitlow often presents tenderness and swelling. The affected area will still be soft despite the swelling. Fever and swelling of the lymph nodes in the upper arm and armpit may also be present.

Conventional Medical Treatment: Staphylococcal whitlow can be treated with antibiotics, rest and elevation of the finger. Moist heat can be applied to aid drainage of pus. Severe cases that present tight swelling of the finger tip may require incision and drainage. Herpetic whitlow can be treated with antiviral medication. Incision and drainage is not recommended. Painkillers can be taken in both instances for pain.

Prognosis: If treated early complications are rare in both types of whitlow. If treatment is delayed or the person is immunocompromised tissue necrosis, osteomyelitis and septic arthritis can occur in staphylococcal whitlow. In herpetic whitlow the infection can be spread to the eyes. There is also risk of scarring and increased sensitivity or numbness in the affected finger.

Holistic Advice: Rest and elevate the affected finger. Cover and avoid touching the affected finger in herpetic whitlow.

Xanthomas

Definition: Soft yellow bumps on the skin caused by accumulation of fat. Xanthelasma are the most common type.

Possible Causes: Most commonly caused by disorders of fat metabolism such as hypercholesterolemia. Diabetes and liver disease can also cause xanthomas to appear. Obesity is a risk factor for developing this condition.

General Signs and Symptoms: Begin as small bumps that enlarge over time, xanthomas are often soft, yellow or yellow-orange in colour. The most common type, xanthelasma, occur on the upper and lower eyelids. Other types of xanthoma can appear on the between the finger/toes, creases of the wrist, elbows, knees, heels and around the Achilles tendon.

Conventional Medical Treatment: Dependent on the cause. Many types of xanthoma will resolve by themselves following treatment of the underlying medical condition. Xanthelasma often improve but not completely disappear. In these cases topical creams, cryotherapy and laser treatments can be used to remove them.

Prognosis: Dependent on the successful treatment and management of the underlying medical condition.

Holistic Advice: Lose weight if required.

Additional Terms

Adhesions – Fibrous bands, often referred to as scar tissue, that occur in the soft tissues (muscle, tendons, ligaments) after microtrauma, overuse or injury.

Allergy – An allergy is an inappropriate immune response, called an allergic reaction, to a normally harmless substance, called an allergen. On initial exposure to the allergen the immune system becomes sensitized to it and produces antibodies. During subsequent exposures, the antibodies produced in response to the allergen bind to the surface of mast cells. Mast cells contain histamine, a substance that causes an inflammatory response, irritating the body tissues and producing the symptoms of an allergic reaction. The mast cells are destroyed by the combination of the antibodies and the allergen, and histamine is released into the body. Common allergic disorders include asthma, eczema and hay fever.

Fainting – A sudden temporary loss of consciousness that often results in a fall. It is caused by a reduced supply of blood and oxygen to the brain and can be caused by neurological or cardiovascular reasons. The feeling of faintness is symptomatic of many conditions such as diabetes, anaemia, heart disease, pregnancy, hypotension and psychological shock.

Fever – Abnormally high temperature. The normal temperature for an adult is between 36 and 36.8°C (96.8 and 98.24°F). Any temperature of 38°C (100.4°F) or above is considered high and is classed as a fever. A fever can be symptomatic of many conditions. If an adult has a temperature above 39°C medical attention should be sought. If a child has a temperature above 39°C urgent medical attention may be required, particularly if the child is unresponsive. Measures such as drinking plenty of cold fluids and lying in a cool room with a free flow of fresh air can help to bring the temperature down.

Female Frigidity – Failure of the woman to respond to a sexual stimulus. It was once believed that the main causes of infertility were impotence in men and frigidity in women. Now that medical knowledge has moved on, many reasons for infertility are appreciated. The reasons for a general lack of interest in sex may be physical, emotional, hormonal or psychological.

Hyperventilation – Increased breathing rate caused by the oxygen level in the body falling too low. Possible causes include asthma, carbon monoxide poisoning, heat exhaustion, heat stroke and hyperglycaemia.

Hysterectomy – Surgical removal of the uterus, and possibly surrounding tissues such as the cervix, fallopian tubes, ovaries, vagina, lymph glands and fatty tissues. Hysterectomies are performed to treat conditions such as endometriosis, menorrhagia (heavy periods), chronic pelvic pain, fibroids and cancer of the ovaries, uterus, cervix or fallopian tubes. It is a major operation with a long recovery period and is only usually considered if less invasive treatments have been ineffective or are not possible.

Intermittent claudication - Medical term for a painful ache in the legs when fatty deposits in the arteries restrict blood flow to the leg muscles. Usually occurs because of atherosclerosis causing peripheral arterial disease.

Muscle Fatigue – The decreased ability of the muscles to contract efficiently over time. The most common cause of muscle fatigue is exercise but conditions such as Addison's disease, fibromyalgia, anaemia and hypothyroidism all have muscle fatigue as a possible symptom. In many cases, muscle fatigue will improve with rest, recovery and hydration.

Muscle Spasm – A sudden involuntary movement in one or more muscles. Most often occur due to stress, exercise or dehydration and can affect any muscle of the body. Muscle spasms can be painful but are very unlikely to be a cause for concern and will resolve by themselves. Trapped nerves and neurological disorders can also cause muscle spasms.

Microtrauma – Very small, often unnoticeable, injuries to the body. Microtrauma can occur anywhere in the body is usually described in the muscles, ligaments, tendons and bones though calluses on the hands and bruised toenails can also be a result. Lifting weights is an example of positive microtrauma in the soft tissue where recovery and remodelling can lead to an increase in size and strength. Repetitive microtrauma can lead to injury or chronic conditions.

Oedema – Fluid retention in the tissues, causing a swelling in the affected area. It can be caused by a variety of factors such as high salt intake in the diet, hot weather, high altitudes, skin burns or being immobile for long periods of time. Oedema is commonly caused by lymphodema. Oedema can also be a symptom of many underlying conditions such as pregnancy, kidney disease, heart failure, chronic lung disease, thyroid disease, liver disease, diabetes, arthritis and malnutrition. When the legs are affected it could be caused by a blood clot, varicose veins or a growth or cyst.

Overuse – Sustained microtrauma from repetitive movements. This can lead to injuries described as overuse injuries. Examples of overuse injuries include repetitive strain injury, carpal tunnel syndrome, bursitis, tendonitis, plantar fasciitis, shin splints, stress fractures, tennis and golfer's elbow.

Pacemaker – A small battery operated device that is implanted in the chest to help the heart beat regularly. Pacemakers are used as a treatment for some heart disorders in which the heart's electrical conducting system is faulty. Cardiac pacemakers stimulate the heart with electrical impulses. Some produce impulses continually, others only send an impulse when the heart rate falls too low. Defibrillator pacemakers send a shock to the heart when the ventricles of the heart are contracting in a rapid or uncoordinated manner. The shock given restores the normal heart rate and rhythm.

Pain – An unpleasant sensation often felt as a result of tissue damage or disease. It usually functions as a warning system that can help to prevent further damage. The location of the pain often acts as a good guide to its source but in some cases pain can be felt in different parts of the body from the site where it originates. This is called referred pain. Referred pain occurs when the nerves carrying the sensation of pain merge with other nerves before they reach the brain.

Palpitations – Heart beats that suddenly become noticeable. The heart may feel as if it is pounding, fluttering or beating irregularly. This may last for just a few seconds or minutes. Sensations may also be felt in the throat or neck. Palpitations may be alarming, but in most cases they are harmless and not a sign of any problem with the heart. Palpitations are most often caused by stimulants, such as caffeine and nicotine, or by anxiety. They may occur as a side effect of some medicines but can be symptomatic of an underlying disorder. If palpitations are frequent or persistent medical attention should be sought, particularly if accompanied by any other symptoms such as shortness of breath, chest pains, feeling faint or fainting.

Paralysis – The loss of ability to move one or more muscles and the loss of sensation in the affected area. It is usually caused by problems with the nerves that control the muscles and so is symptomatic of many nervous system conditions such as stroke, spinal cord injury and multiple sclerosis.

Phlebitis – Literally means inflammation of a vein. Inflamed veins are associated with blood clots. See superficial thrombophlebitis and deep vein thrombosis.

Rheumatism – Is an old fashioned word and nowadays is not the name of an actual condition. Instead it is used as a group reference for the many "rheumatic diseases", which involve inflammation of the joints and connective tissues, e.g. rheumatoid arthritis, tendonitis, bursitis and lupus.

Spastic Colon – Another name for irritable bowel syndrome.

Synovitis – Inflammation of a synovial membrane. It causes joint tenderness, pain and lumps. It is a symptom of several conditions including arthritis, lupus and gout.

Thrombus - A blood clot that is attached to a blood vessel wall, reducing or blocking blood flow. Blood clotting is regulated by chemical reactions between blood cells (platelets) and proteins (clotting factors). Smoking, high stress levels, being overweight/obese, having an unhealthy diet (high in cholesterol) and being inactive can cause clots to form more easily. Conditions such as cancer and diabetes can also increase the risk of clots forming. Atherosclerosis can greatly increase the risk of these clots blocking the arteries/veins, leading to serious conditions such as stroke, heart attack and pulmonary embolism.